MW00791820

AGE LATER

AGE LATER

HEALTH SPAN, LIFE SPAN, AND THE NEW SCIENCE OF LONGEVITY

NIR BARZILAI, M.D.

with Toni Robino

THORNDIKE PRESS
A part of Gale, a Cengage Company

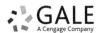

GALE
A Cengage Company

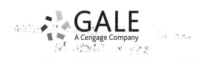

Copyright © 2020 by Nir Barzilai.
Thorndike Press, a part of Gale, a Cengage Company.

Thorndike Press® Large Print Nonfiction.
The text of this Large Print edition is unabridged.
Other aspects of the book may vary from the original edition.
Set in 16 pt. Plantin.

LIBRARY OF CONGRESS CIP DATA ON FILE.
CATALOGUING IN PUBLICATION FOR THIS BOOK
IS AVAILABLE FROM THE LIBRARY OF CONGRESS.

ISBN-13: 978-1-4328-8479-6 (hardcover alk. paper)

Published in 2021 by arrangement with St. Martin's Publishing

Printed in Mexico
Print Number: 01   Print Year: 2021

To my parents and grandparents, who could not age later, and to my wife, Laura, who keeps me young.

CONTENTS

INTRODUCTION 13

One: One Hundred Years Young . . . 23
    The Mysteries of Aging 28
    What Makes SuperAgers Stay
        Healthy? 33
    Studying Centenarians 37
    Designing a Study Without a
        Control Group 48
    Meeting Our First AJ Centenarians
        and Their Offspring 52
    A Perfect Genome?. 56
    Centenarians' Interactions with
        Their Environments 58
    Do as I Say, Not as I Do 70

Two: Why We Age 74
    Recent Theories 83
    The Search for Protection from
        Aging 90
    Eating Less May Lead to More
        Healthy Years 97
    Unlocking the Secrets in Fat . . . 99
    Caloric Restriction: A Mixed Bag
        of Effects 109
    Aging Begins Before We're
        Born 114
    SuperAgers' Top Secrets 115
Three: Cholesterol: Is More
Better? 119
    Unlocking Cholesterol's Longevity
        Secrets 124
    Are There Really Good Gene
        Mutations?. 129
    Solving the Mystery of Helpful
        Gene Mutations. 132
    The Benefits of CETP
        Personified 140
    A Mutation That Adds Years to
        Life Span?. 146

Four: Growth Hormone: Less Is
    More 149
    Less Growth May Lead to an
        Exceptionally Long Life 151
    Growth Hormone Clues from
        Our Centenarians 154
    Epigenetic Mechanisms Can
        Increase Longevity. 163
    Making the Most of Our
        Findings 169
    Growth Hormones Don't "Grow"
        Life Span 173
Five: Unraveling the Longevity
    Mystery Deep Inside Our
    Cells. 177
    A Match Made on Earth. 178
    Mitochondria's Hidden
        Purpose. 180
    Resilient to the End 187
    A CohBar Is Born 198
    Searching for Promising
        Peptides 204

Six: The Quest to Prove Aging Can
    Be Targeted 209
    Choosing an Existing Drug to
       Prove Our Point. 220
    Getting the FDA on Board . . . 225
    How the TAME Study Works . . 228
    Who's Going to Pay for All
       of This?. 235
    Metformin Is the Tool, Not
       the Goal 241
Seven: Making Eighty the New
    Sixty. 245
    The Price of Progress 253
    Collaboration Is the Key to
       Speed 254
    Long, Healthy Life Span Versus
       Immortality. 258
    The Gap Between Making Drugs
       and Making Drugs Available . . 265

Eight: Stop the Clock 268
How Old Is Old? 271
Use It or Lose It 275
Antioxidants and Hormesis . . . 279
Thriving in the Shadow of
    Stress 282
Preventing the Loss of Muscle
    Mass as We Age 288
Exercise Plus Metformin 289
Feeding Our Longevity 291
Hydrating Wisely 297
Prevent Obesity. 299
Nutraceuticals Are in the
    Works 305
The Magic Pills We've Been
    Wishing For 310
When We Eat Matters 313
Our DNA Has Something
    to Say 321
Stay Mentally Sharp 326
Other Promising Practices 336
How to Decide What's Good
    for You 341

11

Nine: Bright Horizons 343
    The Unparalleled Power of
       Omics 344
    Personalized Medicine 350
    Advances in Early Detection . . . 352
    Pioneering Explorations 354
    Reversing Cellular Age 358
    Genetic Engineering 360

ACKNOWLEDGMENTS 363

INTRODUCTION

It was a warm summer day in 1968, and a breeze rippled the leaves on the trees that lined Panorama Street as my grandfather Dov and I walked to the top of Mount Carmel, where we could see Haifa Bay. Across the bay were the Galilee mountains, Nazareth, and Golan Heights. I was thirteen and Grandfather was sixty-eight, and we walked this route nearly every Saturday as he told me stories about his life. My sisters and I were born in Haifa and grew up there, as did our father, so many of the stories' settings were familiar to me. On this day, he told me the story of planting trees on the roads to Jerusalem and draining swamps in Hadera. I idolized him and hung on his every word as he explained the challenges involved and the strength required to accomplish those tasks.

Each of his stories made him seem larger than life — strong, active, unwavering. But

13

as we crested the hill, he was breathing heavily and leaned over, placing his hands on his thighs as if he might topple over. I stood watching him, wondering if there was something I should do to help him. I'd never seen him so out of breath. *How could this slow, overweight man — balding and wrinkled — be the man from the stories? How could he plant trees and drain swamps and build businesses? How could that person have become* this *person?*

Grandfather continued his story a minute later, but that moment sparked the first of the great mysteries in my life, one that ultimately helped push me into medicine and has tantalized me for decades. Aging transforms us, remakes us, breaks us, destroys us. But why?

I'm still asking that question, and as I near the age my grandfather was on that memorable day, my quest has taken on new meaning. My grandfather died of a heart attack at age sixty-eight, but thanks to improvements that have been made in medical interventions over the past hundred years, my father, David, who had a heart attack at the same age, underwent triple bypass surgery and lived another two decades. And preventive measures have improved so much that *I'm* planning to skip the heart attack altogether.

For thousands of years before the twentieth century, most people died between the ages of twenty-five and thirty-five. Forty years old was considered ancient. Of course, there were always exceptions, and we know that some people, like Leonardo da Vinci and Rembrandt, lived to be very old, but it wasn't until the twentieth century that life expectancy for men and women exceeded sixty years, thanks to sanitation, immunizations, antibiotics, medication, surgery, and other innovations. By the mid-1900s, human life span increased until the average reached eighty years, which is where we are now. But we start accumulating diseases after the age of sixty, and many people are being treated for three different diseases or chronic conditions by the age of seventy-five. So regarding the future of humanity and quality of life, it's clear that finding a way to prevent or delay the onset of age-related illnesses is one of the most important mysteries we can solve. I have dedicated my life to this quest, not just because of the vision I have for the future but also because of some lessons from my past.

When I was a medical student at the Israeli Institute of Technology, I was also a medic and a nurse, so I wanted to use my

15

knowledge and skills to help wherever they were needed most. My first opportunity was during the winter of 1979/80 when Vietnam invaded Cambodia and overthrew the oppressive regime of Pol Pot and his "killing fields." I was one of ten people on the Israeli government mission team that traveled to the border of Cambodia and Thailand to work in the Sakeo refugee camp under the auspices of the Red Cross. These refugees, many of whom had been soldiers under Pol Pot's rule, were dying of the same things that have afflicted humankind since the beginning of our existence — namely, infectious disease, starvation, and violent conflict with other humans. We saved thousands of lives, but for each one we saved, another dozen died. Despite this nightmare, all the volunteers worked relentlessly, including the Salvation Army missionaries, who had set up a small shelter in the middle of camp where children could have a drink and a snack while the volunteers told them Bible stories. So everyone was offering whatever skills and services we could provide, and eventually, we made some progress by keeping more of the refugees alive.

But we also saw many people die before they had a chance to grow old, and that had a lasting impact on me and gave me a deeper appreciation for life. It also made me think of how fortunate my grandfather had been to live so long even though his last years were not healthy. And the question was sparked again: Why can't we live long *and* be healthy?

My time working in the Cambodian refugee camp also taught me something that empowered me to keep searching for the answer to that question. This unexpected lesson came to me by way of three Buddhist monks who approached me one day as I was in the storage shed, looking for supplies. They greeted me with their hands clasped in prayer, two middle-aged men wearing yellow gowns and an older man wearing orange. He spoke fluent English but surprised me by saying, "Shalom," and other Hebrew words. He said he was the Tana-Jan, the high Buddhist priest for large areas of Cambodia, Thailand, and Laos, and he invited me and other members of the Israeli team to his temple to discuss a problem of grave importance.

That night, four of us and a guide traveled what felt like a very long way to the temple. But when the guide stopped the van, all we could see was a narrow path that led into the jungle. He instructed us to stay close behind him, and we walked through the dense foliage in the dimming light. The sounds that the birds and other animals in the jungle were making were unfamiliar and intimidating, but our guide pressed on until we finally reached a clearing and a small, one-story temple made of wood.

The Tana-Jan welcomed us and invited us inside. The room was huge and mostly empty, but on the bookshelves were many foreign-language dictionaries, books written in Latin, and books on Islam and Christianity. I was surprised to see that there were also Hebrew books and books about Judaism. He invited us to meditate with him, and while we were unable to reach his level of tranquility, as physicians, we were most impressed by his unnaturally low pulse rate (which we could measure by looking at the pulsation of the carotid artery in his neck). After meditation, the Tana-Jan explained that he had decided to speak to "the chosen people" about his distress. I had thought he had a medical question, but that was not the case. He explained that he was concerned that the missionary action of the Salvation Army would lead Buddhist children in the camp to convert to Christianity for the small gift of drink and food. He felt that these distressed youths were not able to make decisions based on free choice. He

18

thought that as Jews, we could negotiate between the Christians and the Buddhists and stop what he perceived to be a disaster.

I was surprised and overwhelmed by his request. All of a sudden, I questioned whether Major Eva's well-intentioned efforts were appropriate. But at the same time, I'd witnessed how comforting religious beliefs were to those who were sick and had lost loved ones or were facing death themselves. So I thought that if there were a place in the camp for the refugees to practice their own religion, that could promote their well-being.

We returned to the camp the next morning and negotiated a deal with the Red Cross administrator of the camp. Next to the Salvation Army shed, a shed for the Buddhist followers was to be erected. Children would still get food and drink, but they could choose which shed to go to. As it worked out, after that second shed was built, we saw children and other refugees in both places. Coming from the Middle East, where religious conflict has been a cause of wars and misery, I felt that facilitating peace between two religious groups was one of the most significant contributions we could make to the refugees because peace allows for healing, reparation, and life.

Solving the conflict between the Christians and the Buddhists at the refugee camp is one of the experiences that taught me that I could set goals that some may think are unattainable and achieve great things with help from others and a little bit of luck. Without this knowledge, I may not have thought to take on the uphill battle to prove that the hallmarks of aging can be targeted to delay aging and its diseases. While I was full of hope when I began my journey into the biology of aging, very few people shared my enthusiasm, and many people thought that my goal was unachievable. Early studies provided clues that were encouraging, though, and within a decade, the new field of geroscience was thriving, and my colleagues and I have shown through a variety of research studies that aging can, in fact, be targeted. Today, we're focused on making this knowledge applicable for the general public by exploring and developing new treatments and drugs that target the causes of aging.

My journey parallels the evolution of this discovery. Along the way, I've studied animal models and discovered mechanisms for exceptional longevity in humans. To shorten the time line between research and human application, I have also taken on a leadership role in solving the challenges involved with proving that targeting aging can prevent an array of age-related diseases.

In a very short period of time, geroscientists have revolutionized the discipline: to think of aging not as a certainty but as a phenomenon — like many other difficult conditions — that can be targeted, improved, and even cured as if it were a disease. To that end, we are creating biotech companies and other ventures so that as soon as our nationwide double-blind human clinical trial produces the evidence needed by the FDA, more treatments, new drugs, and combinations of drugs that slow aging and increase health span will become available.

After decades of direct research as well as nationwide and worldwide collaborative projects that brought previously isolated researchers together, we are finally able to say that aging, as we know it, is over.

ONE:
ONE HUNDRED YEARS YOUNG

Have you heard the one about the woman who asked her eighty-year-old husband, "Want to go upstairs and make love?"

"I'm sorry, honey," he said. "I can't do both."

In the near future, the punch line may not work. Having overcome these limitations, we will be enjoying a new reality of being healthy and vital in our nineties and beyond. We are on the leading edge of a revolution that will dramatically change the way we age. It may sound like science fiction, but I promise you it's *science.* To be exact, it's geroscience, an interdisciplinary field that studies the relationship between aging and age-related diseases. This collaboration has built a bridge between the interests of biologists exploring the basic mechanisms that drive aging and geriatricians trying to improve elderly patients' quality of life. And I'm delighted to report that the future is

23

very bright.

This new reality is made possible by what we're learning from centenarians like the Kahn siblings — Irving, Helen, Peter, and Leonore. The four children had been born during the first decade of the twentieth century, when the average life expectancy at birth was only forty years. They'd seen each other through wars, deaths, and divorces and celebrated together at the birth of grandchildren and great-grandchildren. Leonore and Helen had joined the first Girl Scout troop in New York, and as an adult, Leonore became a troop leader and trained volunteers for more than fifty years. Helen enjoyed a long career as a magazine writer, which she began in 1936. Peter was a cameraman on such movies as *Gone with the Wind* and *The Wizard of Oz* and a photographer with Frank Capra in the Pacific theater of World War II. He also helped to develop Technicolor and worked in video technology at HBO until retiring at eighty-one. Irving first went to work on Wall Street in 1928, before the Great Depression. Everything imaginable had changed over the course of their lives, but in a physical sense, time seemed to be standing still for these four siblings.

Yes, they'd aged. But the changes we associate with aging — lost mobility, lost intellect, lost excitement, lost energy — had been delayed for decades. They lived more than two and a half times as long as most of their peers, and instead of declining, they each continued to thrive. Leonore was still giving tours at an environmental learning center well into her nineties. Irving continued to work at the family investment firm at 108, bossing around his son and grandson who also worked there. Peter remarried at seventy-three and was happy with his new wife for more than thirty years. Helen drank Budweiser, went to Manhattan museums and trendy restaurants, and smoked for more than ninety years.

That's what makes the Kahns so extraordinary. They weren't eating anything special, exercising outside their daily routines, drinking extra water, napping, or doing anything else that we tend to think of as healthy, life-extending habits. They didn't strive to keep their bodies whole and their minds nimble — they just, somehow, *were.*

Like many centenarians, the Kahns simply aged more slowly than most of the population — meaning they, in effect, *aged later.* But why? That's the question I've been studying for almost two decades, and I have encouraging news. Scientific advances are making the sandwich generation a thing of the past. Instead of being pulled in two directions by needing to care for our aging parents while we raise our children, we can watch our healthy parents play active roles in their grandchildren's lives.

Later in the book, you'll learn more about Irving Kahn, along with some of our other centenarians, including:

- Ervin Adam, ninety-seven, my uncle and one of the most resilient people I have ever known. After surviving six concentration camps during World War II and fleeing Czechoslovakia as the Soviets invaded in 1968, he bounced back *again* after losing everything to Hurricane Harvey in 2017. And after finally retiring from the Baylor College of Medicine at ninety-four, he still attends lectures every week.
- My wife's grandmother Frieda, another centenarian who defied the medical texts. Remarkably active and determined to keep enjoying life, she broke her ankle at age one hundred, and she insisted on having surgery even though her doctor thought a wheelchair would be a safer option.

And this new frontier isn't just exciting from the standpoint of slowing aging and the onset of disease — it also has other profound implications. People who undergo chemotherapy or radiation treatment age rapidly, and that places them at higher risk for another disease or a second cancer. And the children who survive after having these treatments start having age-related diseases, such as hypertension and cardiovascular disease, at much younger ages than we see in the general population. These people desperately need our help, as do people with HIV. The treatment they receive to survive may be aging them faster than the virus, and on average, they get all the age-related diseases about ten years sooner than people who do not have HIV. Another large group of people who need interventions against rapid aging are those with physical disabilities and permanent injuries who cannot exercise as much as others can and tend to become obese, which accelerates aging. All these people can benefit from the new treatments and drugs that are being developed, so targeting the causes of aging truly benefits many more groups than the elderly. And the benefits of these new developments even extend beyond our sick and suffering. They will be vitally important in our quest to reach new frontiers, on the planet and off. When astronauts make the voyage to Mars, they will be exposed to radiation for years, and the discoveries we make with genetic testing and research will also lead to revolutionary approaches to protecting people when they leave Earth's atmosphere.

THE MYSTERIES OF AGING

We can understand why the circle of life includes death, but *aging* is different. Why would an organism evolve to deteriorate as it grows older? How does it benefit us as a species to have eyesight dwindle, mobility decline, stamina evaporate, bones wither, and bellies get bigger? As a scientist and a gerontologist, I assure you that these losses and indignities no longer need to define the last decades of our lives. When we ask people in the United States how long they want to live, they usually say between seventy-nine and a hundred years, and in one study, the median number of years was ninety, but those responses are influenced by the effects of old age that people have witnessed, and the past does not dictate the future. An average U.S. life span of eighty-nine is just the current norm. When people can live beyond one hundred while maintaining their faculties and enjoying good health, we might feel shortchanged if we only make it to ninety-five.

Growing old may seem as normal as growing up, but when we look closer, we see that it's a complex and often painful mystery. And it's a mystery we must solve because aging poses a dramatic increase in our risk of having every chronic disease. The major risk for *all* types of cancer is aging, and so is the major risk for diabetes and Alzheimer's. We have a hundred- to thousand-fold greater chance of dying from aging than of dying from other risks like obesity or high cholesterol.

Everyone talks about cholesterol contributing to cardiovascular disease, but it's only a threefold risk, whereas aging is a thousandfold risk for dying from cardiovascular disease. Cardiologists have argued that cardiovascular disease is just accumulation of plaque over time, but we know from autopsies of people in their twenties that plaque can start to form early on. For the first forty or fifty years of our lives, we can deal with those plaques, and they are actually dynamic — forming and going away. After age fifty, we start to lose the ability to control plaque accumulation because some of the biological processes that controlled it, decline. Some evidence suggests that a

29

series of changes or mutations makes an organism likelier to die from loss of cells or from cancer, other evidence suggests it's an increase in inflammation levels or oxidative damage that causes aging, and still other results suggest that aging occurs when our bodies lose the ability to activate the stem cells that keep our other cells healthy. All these theories have merit, but none of them alone is enough. To the degree that they're true, they all drive aging together.

Most chronic diseases are united by one primary cause — the biology of *aging itself*. While there are genetic and environmental bases for many age-related diseases, aging increases our chances of contracting them more than any other factor alone. Aging is the main reason for the global epidemic of chronic diseases. The World Health Organization (WHO) estimates that these age-related diseases are responsible for about 70 percent of the global death rate and 80 percent of U.S. Medicare costs, which the WHO projects will cost the global economy more than $30 trillion by 2030. While life expectancy in the United States ranges from 74.7 years for West Virginians to 81.3 years for Hawaiians, research shows that the average American enjoys only 67.7 *healthy* years. So nobody can logically argue that we don't need to accelerate our ability to increase health span — the span of good health. But based on health-adjusted life expectancy (HALE), the United States is not doing well with this. In fact, we're doing worse than the European Union and ten other countries ranked in a report by the Aging Analytics Agency, coming in dead last after China. The three-hundred-page report points out that this is despite the fact that, among developed countries, the United States spends the most on health care per capita, at $9,892. Unfortunately, that number is predicted to grow an average of 5.5 percent a year through 2026, and if that happens, by 2027, health care spending will represent 19.4 percent of gross domestic product.

If we don't make some dramatic changes in how we approach health and instead continue to treat one disease at a time, the best we can hope for is exchanging one disease for another. Making matters worse, these age-related diseases tend to accumulate and lead to functional decline. Often, surviving one onslaught only buys time for another onslaught. We've all heard about someone who had a stent installed or had coronary bypass surgery to prevent a heart attack and then died from a different chronic disease a few years later. Treating one disease at a time or targeting just one organ rather than targeting aging is a miserable approach — and it's not working. When I started on the quest to understand aging, most of the research had been focused on the causes of aging, so I decided to approach the problem from the opposite side and find out what delays it.

When I entered the field, scientists like George Martin, one of the fathers of modern gerontology and a mentor to me, were trying to solve the mystery of aging predominantly by studying children with progeria, rare syndromes that age people far faster than what is considered normal — in effect, their biological age races ahead of their chronological age. But although those studies were extensive, the findings didn't unlock many secrets of aging. So I thought that instead of studying people who age rapidly, we would study centenarians — those lucky folks who appear to be far healthier and more youthful than their years would predict. Centenarians are extraordinary because even as their chronological age ticks relentlessly forward, their biological age hangs years or even decades behind.

Studying centenarians led us to ask many questions, but the biggest one was:

Can we prevent or delay aging?

The answer is *yes.*

We still have a lot to learn, but the promise I can make is that help is on the way, thanks in part to the secrets of "SuperAgers" like the centenarians in our studies at the Albert Einstein College of Medicine's Institute for Aging Research, which I founded. For them, the outlook is entirely different — all the chronic diseases are delayed. We experience old age and illness as one and the same thing, whether it's diabetes or Alzheimer's, Parkinson's or cancer, but at seventy, the SuperAgers have twenty to thirty more mostly disease-free years ahead of them. My research team and I are on a mission to find out how these people are living such long lives in such remarkable health. Each time we unlock one of their secrets, we explore how we can use what we learned to benefit everyone else.

WHAT MAKES SUPERAGERS STAY HEALTHY?

Many centenarians pass the hundred-year mark almost effortlessly. Whereas most people are ill for an average of five to eight years prior to death, centenarians tend to maintain most of their abilities and are ill for only about five to eight months before their deaths. While we expected many of the centenarians we studied to be diagnosed with cardiovascular disease, Alzheimer's, and Parkinson's at higher percentages, they weren't. That said, it's important to clarify that centenarians' bodies are not young. Many of them have some limitations like poor eyesight or hearing, some have less mobility than others, and arthritis is common. But the major diseases are delayed, and at the age of their retirement, many of them were not seeing a doctor and had no medical expenses. Surprisingly, the health care costs of the average person who lives past one hundred are only 30 percent of those of the average person who dies in their seventies.

Studying SuperAgers, people who are still living independently by age ninety-five, based on their DNA and other biological factors, is central to understanding the blueprint for how we all can age more slowly and maintain our good health. By discovering what makes these people so special, we're discovering the real secrets of aging for the first time. SuperAgers largely sidestep the diseases that plague their peers — diabetes, cognitive decline, cardiovascular disease, Alzheimer's, and cancer — main-

THE ABCS OF DNA AND RNA

DNA — deoxyribonucleic acid — is a molecule made up of two chains (a.k.a. polynucleotides) that carry the genetic instructions for growth, development, functioning, and reproduction of living organisms and many viruses.

RNA — ribonucleic acid — is a large molecule essential to the coding, decoding, regulation, and expression of genes.

Nucleotides are the building blocks of nucleic acids.

Nucleic acids are the small molecules essential to all forms of life.

Gene expression is the process by which the instructions of the DNA are translated to a protein through "messenger" RNA (mRNA).

The DNA alphabet consists of four letters, each of which represents a type of nucleotide:

A   Adenine
C   Cytosine
G   Guanine
T   Thymine

taining vibrant lives that may slow down but don't dim. They're successful business leaders, musicians, and artists living independently into their late nineties and older. They help to raise their grandchildren, travel the world, learn new skills, and live full lives far longer than the rest of us. When they do contract debilitating diseases, it happens much later in life — sometimes two to three decades later than for most people and for a very compressed period of time.

We might theorize that these people derive all these benefits because they have healthier lifestyles than the rest of us, but that's not the case. Instead, many of them break the health rules that the rest of us need to follow. Nearly 50 percent of the centenarians in our study are overweight or obese, nearly 50 percent smoke, and fewer than 50 percent do even moderate exercise. Remember the Kahns? When I asked Helen, who lived to 110 and smoked for more than ninety years, "Didn't *any* of your doctors tell you to stop smoking?" she said, "Sure, but all four of those doctors died."

Demographers estimate that for most people, genetics are responsible for about 20–25 percent of aging and the environment is responsible for the rest. But the statistics are vastly different for centenarians, whose genes are about 75–80 percent responsible for how they age and the environment accounts for only about 20 percent. That's why we're so determined to unlock their secrets. Doing so can give us insight into providing everyone with the same protections from aging that they enjoy.

Besides being medical marvels, these amazing people have made the most of their "extra years" by remaining engaged with life and dwelling on the positive. Every SuperAger I've met has interesting stories to tell and pearls of wisdom to share, no matter how humble they might be about sharing them. They make me look forward to the day when all our elders can be engaged members of society well into their nineties and beyond. At Einstein, we are determined to make that happen sooner rather than later.

STUDYING CENTENARIANS

The idea to look for the secrets of longevity in centenarians was exciting and promising, but figuring out how to design and conduct the study was devilishly complicated. How could we study a population that had no living control group? And what should we be looking for?

When we started the Longevity Genes

Project in 1998, we had three distinct hypotheses about what made centenarians so special genetically. One was that the centenarians had a perfect genome, one without any variants or other errors or imperfections in the sequence of the genetic code of DNA, allowing them to grow and age in the most optimal way. The second hypothesis was that centenarians had very healthy lifestyles and environments. Our third hypothesis was that centenarians had all the same variants in their DNA as the rest of us but were being protected from their negative effects by *other* variants in the sequence of their DNA. If that was the case, though, how could we discover those protective variants?

Common changes that occur across the DNA in individuals are known as *variants,* some of which are associated with and may cause diseases. If the variants are rare, they're known as *mutations.* Each variant or mutation gets a single nucleotide polymorphic (SNP) number that identifies it in the sequence of the genome.

As for finding answers, strong data suggests that exceptional longevity runs in families — people with a centenarian parent are about ten to twenty times likelier to become a centenarian or have a sibling who

MUTATIONS AND VARIANTS

A mutation is a natural and permanent change in the sequence of the chromosomal DNA. Mutations are rare. Only about one person in one million has a mutation that causes a phenotype of sickness, or for centenarians, extended health.

A variant is a mutation that has spread into the population and therefore has become more common.

Geroscientists are looking at rare and common variants associated with exceptional longevity in our centenarian population.

will make it to one hundred than people who don't have centenarian parents. For that reason, it made sense for us to study exceptional longevity genetically. And because it's rare, it's easier to find genetic differences in a group of centenarians than in a group of people with common illnesses like diabetes or hypertension. When the human genome was sequenced, we looked for common variant differences between people with diseases and people without diseases, but we were disappointed by how little we found. Despite the great expense of the technology at the time, the genetic information we got usually explained less than 5 percent of the contribution that these common variants made to each of the common diseases. This happened because most of the DNA we have is not coding for the genes that make up the less than 30,000 proteins that make up our biology. So about 90 percent of the variants are overrepresented in noncoding areas and underrepresented in the regions that code the exact sequence of a protein. In other words, there are more variants near the genes, between the genes, and between the coding sequences of the genes than in the coding sequences of the genes themselves. We were more interested in finding genetic variants in the coding regions of the genes, but at that time, we knew there was no chance of getting funded because the genetic testing was extremely expensive and had major quality-control issues. Furthermore, to study this in an unbiased way, we needed to design a scientific study that was solid enough to get funding. In particular, we needed to figure out how to isolate what made centenarians genetically different without being able to compare them with their peers who had died decades earlier.

I should point out that by no means was I the first scientist to be interested in centenarians. But in the quest for genuine secrets for health span and longevity, I put together the first group to study centenarians' biology and genetics, and we launched the Longevity Genes Project the year after Madame Jeanne Calment died at the age of 122. Madame Calment, who became a celebrity of sorts, stirred a lot of interest in centenarian studies because she was known for being "young" well into her later years. Calment was born in 1875 in Arles, France, and lived there for her entire life. Arles is known for inspiring Vincent van Gogh's paintings, and Calment met Van Gogh when she was twelve. When she was twenty-one, she married a second cousin and went on to enjoy a prosperous life filled with physical activity, including fencing, swimming, tennis, cycling, and mountaineering. Her husband died in 1942 when she was sixty-seven, but that didn't slow her down. She continued to participate in all the activities she'd enjoyed with her husband for decades, including riding her bike around Arles until she was one hundred. She reportedly ate two pounds of chocolate every day and credited her olive oil–rich diet for her calm disposition and her long life. "That's why they call me *Calme*nt," she used to say. (*Calm* in French is *calme*.)

When she was ninety, a notary by the name of Andre-Francois Raffray made her an offer to buy her apartment, with the condition that she could live there until she died and he would pay her 2,500 francs a month until then. Not only did Calment outlive Raffray, but the payments she'd received amounted to more than twice the apartment's value. "In life, one sometimes makes bad deals," she reportedly said of Raffray's ultimately losing proposition. Calment lived on her own until she moved into a nursing home at age 110, and she remained physically active until she was injured in a fall when she was 115. But even after that, her mind remained sharp.

It is possible that other people have reached age 122, but validating such claims is difficult. I was on a panel that heard the twenty-five pieces of evidence that validated the findings for Madame Calment's age, and you can be sure that the panel was very thorough, because understanding our maximal capacity for life span is essential for aging research. Some disagreed with Calment's claimed age, but in the paper disputing her age that I reviewed, no substantial evidence was provided. One argument was that the physician who saw her on her one hundredth birthday commented that she looked twenty years younger than her age. But at Einstein, we had collaborated with Anne Chang, associate professor of dermatology at Stanford University School of Medicine, on a study of skin-aging genes in which we'd objectively assessed the skin age of our centenarians and found it to be about twenty-four years younger than their chronological age on average. So of course Calment looked younger than her age. I'm certain that the unsubstantiated "conspiracy" theory that she was actually her daughter won't prove out. There's no way that we were off by even a year, let alone two decades.

So, comfortable with using 122 as our high-water mark, I began thinking about which centenarians we should study in the Longevity Genes Project and how to find them. Although the fact that exceptional longevity is rare and tends to run in families makes centenarians a good phenotype — or a set of observable physical characteristics — for genetic studies, this phenotype becomes a disadvantage when it comes to finding enough people nearby to conduct a large study. When we started the study, it

43

was estimated that only one in ten thousand people was a centenarian. Today, the number may be closer to five in ten thousand thanks to life-extending hip and knee replacements, artificial limbs, and pacemakers, but even though their longevity isn't entirely "naturally occurring," you still need some genetic help to make it that far. And while the expanded pool helps some, five people in ten thousand is still a pretty small number.

The Icelandic population is the best population in the world for genetic studies because there are fewer than half a million Icelandics, and they are all descendants of five Viking men and four Irish women — you can't get much more interrelated than that. So the chances of finding genetic differences that account for any disease would be very high in that population compared with the chances of finding them in New York City. Genetically diverse populations create a lot of genetic noise in studies, which makes it more difficult to find genetic causes. But unfortunately, I needed more centenarians than the Icelandic population has, and besides, Iceland is a long commute from the Bronx, where the Einstein Institute is located.

Curious about how many centenarians

were living close by, I checked the records at the voter registration office. At that time, the population of the Bronx was just over six hundred thousand, so I estimated that I could recruit fewer than a hundred centenarians in the borough. Imagine my surprise when I saw that close to five thousand centenarians were living in the Bronx! When I looked closer, I saw that many of them were allegedly 150 years old or older, and I smelled a voting scam. The practice of using the names of dead people to vote is just one example of why it can be hard to verify someone's true age, and the challenge is worldwide. The Japanese are the longest-living people in the world, but some families wait for years before they announce the death of parents so that they can continue to collect social security. So while the average life expectancy is eighty-four for Japan's population, we cannot always trust the reported ages of individuals, in particular when they are so old.

After exploring a few other dead ends, it occurred to me that I should recruit only Ashkenazi Jews (AJs) for the study because of the homogeneity of their population. They have remarkably uniform genetics, which resulted from discrimination, persecution, isolation, inbreeding, and population expansion that followed "bottleneck" periods when many died. For these reasons, their DNA gives us an advantage in identifying genetic diseases. An example of their genetic closeness is the prevalence of Tay-Sachs disease among their population. About 3.5 percent of Ashkenazi Jews in the United States are carriers of the disease, compared with 0.33 percent of the general population. When a particular gene mutation is inherited from one of the parents, the offspring carrying the disease is called *heterozygous* and does not have symptoms of the disease. If a particular gene mutation is inherited from both parents, it's *homozygous* and results in the manifestation of TaySachs. About one in 3,600 Ashkenazi Jews in the United States have the disease, compared with one in 320,000 in the general population. With the advantage of such clearly drawn lines between heterozygosity and homozygosity, we started looking for links between these conditions and longevity.

We don't think Ashkenazi Jews are more or less likely to become centenarians than people in other populations, but we know they share many common ancestors — 40 percent of all Ashkenazi descend from just four mothers, according to markers in the

DNA of their mitochondria (which is almost always inherited from mothers only). Because, like the Icelandic population, they are so genetically close, the sequence of their DNA is less noisy and much easier to study than the DNA of a genetically diverse population. Another factor in our decision was that Ashkenazi Jews in the United States are similar in socioeconomic levels, and we know that education and income have a major influence on health span in this country. Last, most of the Ashkenazi Jews in America live in the New York area and between Boston and Washington, D.C. — places my study could reach more easily than Iceland.

Our first participants in the Longevity Genes Project came to us courtesy of people we knew, and we used passports, birth certificates, and driver's licenses to verify age. Einstein chief of endocrinology Norman Fleischer, who had recruited me to the institute, and his wife, Eva, introduced me to her mother, who was 102. Norman was smart, knowledgeable, and one of the best clinicians I've ever met. He was a dear father figure to me, so it meant a lot to me that he was the one who connected me with one of the first centenarians in the study. Next, Ruth Freeman, a women's health endocrinologist and a great educator, introduced me to her mother and aunt, who were both over the age of one hundred.

After that, word of mouth led us from one centenarian to another, and we were surprised by how many of them knew each other. Then, shortly after we met the Kahn siblings, we started to get publicity, including an extensive article in *New York* magazine, and our numbers started to grow. People called us to say that their relative or neighbor was a centenarian, and we also received help from Jewish homes for the elderly and the Dorot Foundation, a wonderful nonprofit organization that helps to alleviate social isolation and provides services for older adults.

DESIGNING A STUDY WITHOUT A CONTROL GROUP

Figuring out how to set up a control group for the study was another challenge because most of the centenarians' peers had been dead for decades. The first centenarians in our early studies were born between 1895 and 1910, when the average life expectancy was only about forty years because so many people died from childhood diseases. The people who made it to forty had a life expectancy of a little over sixty. So the centenarians lived forty years longer than their friends, who would have been the real control group. For a controlled study, we'd need to compare the DNA of centenarians with the DNA of unrelated people who were born and shared the environment at the same time as they had but had died. Grave digging wasn't an option, so we had to find another way.

And while we looked for it, we also grappled with what we should measure in the centenarians' blood samples. My line of thinking was that analyzing anything but their DNA at that age might be misleading. For example, assume that we're measuring something in the blood of centenarians and we find that they have significantly higher levels than the normal value. On one hand, it could have contributed to their longevity, but on the other hand, since any given centenarian has almost a 30 percent chance of dying in the next twelve months, the high levels could also have been predictors of death.

With those considerations, we decided to recruit not only centenarians but also one offspring of each, because the offspring have half of the longevity genes and the phenotype of their centenarian parent. So if something measures high in centenarians and it's also high in their offspring, it probably has something to do with their longevity. Another benefit of including the offspring is that we can isolate the longevity mutations and track them as they're passed down through the generations. But the most important reason to recruit the offspring is that while we could not create a control group for their parents, we could create one for them.

Initially, the control group was composed of the spouses of the offspring if they were Ashkenazi Jews with all four grandparents being AJs. None of the spouses in the control group had grandparents who had lived longer than age eighty-five, so we knew they didn't have longevity in their families. Since the spouses were part of the homogeneous population, lived in the same house and community as the offspring, and had similar health habits, we determined that they were a valid control group.

Our next step was to submit our plans for the study to the Institutional Review Board (IRB), which protects the rights and welfare of people who participate in research studies. The IRB is responsible for reviewing all proposed research studies that include human participants, and it has the right to approve, disapprove, oversee, and require changes in all research that is under its jurisdiction. So we sent our study proposal to the IRB, and I explained that we would be looking at centenarians and their children. The next day, the proposal was back on my desk with a note: "For children, you need different forms." But of course, we were talking about eighty-year-old children, and we decided that the term *offspring* would probably cause less confusion.

Today, the control group consists mostly of AJs who are neighbors of the centenarians' offspring rather than spouses. We included these people in the control group because the reviewers of our grants were concerned about assortative mating, which refers to a pattern of choosing mates in which people with similar traits and habits mate more frequently than we'd expect (under a random mating pattern). An obese person is likelier to marry an obese person, a vegetarian is likelier to mate with a vegetarian, and a smoker is likelier to marry a smoker. This tendency carries over into income and education levels, too. In the United States and to a lesser extent in other countries, when you marry, you choose a lot of the health issues that you may have later. We thought mates made a better control group than neighbors, because mates share the same environment and tend to have similar habits and diets (although, granted, one could certainly eat significantly more than the other). And we argued that spouses of the centenarians' offspring didn't marry them based on the longevity of their parents. For one thing, their parents weren't centenarians when the offspring married, so they didn't have that information at the time. But we rolled with the punches and recruited neighbors in addition to the mates, and our data shows that the two control subgroups are genetically similar.

MEETING OUR FIRST AJ CENTENARIANS AND THEIR OFFSPRING

I met with the first several centenarians myself, and one of the questions I asked them was whether exceptional longevity ran in their families. It turned out that it usually did, with many of them saying they had family members who had lived to be one hundred or older. This supported our theory that exceptional longevity is primarily based on genetics, and so did the centenarians themselves. When asked why they think they live longer, their number-one response was genetics. None of this surprised us, though, because Tom Perls, director of the New

England Centenarian Study at Boston University, Paola Sebastiani, genetics professor, and other investigators had already shown that exceptional longevity is often inherited.

Besides talking at length with the first centenarians, I examined them and took their blood. By the time the study was officially under way, I had used that information to create a questionnaire adapted from one that had been validated in large studies, but trying to figure out what to ask before that questionnaire was in place provided some challenges. For example, colleagues and friends had all sorts of ideas about what I should ask, but an overwhelming number of them thought there was a connection between longevity and napping. So I added napping to my list of questions, and the next time I interviewed a centenarian, I asked him if he napped.

"I nap every afternoon," he said.

Wow, I thought, *we might be onto something.* "Did you nap every day last year, too?"

He thought about it. "No."

"How about the year before that?"

He shook his head. "I don't think so. I don't remember. But I remember taking naps the year I retired."

If he had retired a few years before this conversation, that might have been an indication of a pattern, but he'd retired more than twenty years earlier. So while centenarians may have once had habits that contributed to their longevity, we cannot rely on their memories to be accurate, and their habits may have changed from year to year. But we *can* rely on our lab results and the health histories that we take when we meet each centenarian and one offspring.

Meeting the centenarians quickly became a highlight of my work. I could easily sit with them all day to hear their stories, insights, and wisdom, carried from my grandparents' generation. Many members of that generation were Holocaust survivors, including my uncle Ervin, who suffered in six different concentration camps before World War II ended. Ever since I was a young boy, I was impressed by stories about my uncle Ervin, as well as the stories he told me about my family that my mother — another survivor — wouldn't talk about. Now here I was listening to the stories of other people who were part of the same generation and had experienced some of the same events. They all made indelible impressions on me, but the commonalities I shared with Benjamin were especially moving. At

104, Benjamin was alert, charming, and thoughtful. He had been born in 1898 in a tiny settlement in Israel called Rishon LeZion. Settled by Russian Jews, it was the second Jewish farm settlement in Israel. When I met him in 2002 in New Jersey, he said the settlement was located not far from Sarafand al-Amar, where the British army had built the biggest transportation base in the Middle East.

"Sarafand?" I asked.

He nodded.

"That's where I served!"

He had served with the British army, and I had served more than fifty years later with the Israeli army, and we discovered we'd even lived in the same barracks. For Benjamin, having a job as a truck driver at the base and being able to live in the barracks had been a godsend. For me, the time I spent at Sarafand had also been a godsend, though in a very different way. Over the course of the three years I spent with the Israeli Medical Corps in the 1970s, I progressed from a medic to an instructor of medics to a chief medic to the army's chief medical officer. I went from bunking with fifty other soldiers to having my own office, car, and secretary and doing inspections by helicopter. A lifetime career in three years.

I realized that the man pouring coffee across the kitchen table from me not only had had a life that preceded the state of Israel but had also been born before radio broadcasting, penicillin, and air travel. And because he had endured and continued to thrive, our lives were now intertwined. He was a pharmacist and I a doctor, both of us living outside New York City, both of us far from our original homes. How much we had to say to each other and learn from each other. Nothing separated our stories but time, and as we talked, a century contracted to the size of the kitchen table. *This,* I thought, *this is what it should be like to age. We should all be so lucky!*

With that goal in mind, it was time to start testing some hypotheses.

A PERFECT GENOME?

In light of the disappointing results we got from the very expensive process of human genome sequencing, we decided to focus on the genes that we thought were the best candidates to be involved in aging. To create a list of these "candidate genes," we measured several blood components in families of centenarians and found out about their biology. With gene sequencing, we could find out if any of the centenarians' variants we found differed from the variants of members of an unrelated control group.

To test the hypothesis that centenarians had a perfect genome, we conducted the entire genome sequencing in our first forty-four centenarians. After performing the sequencing, which consists of reading the sequence of approximately 3.2 billion nucleotides that make up the genome of each individual, we obtained information from a database called ClinVar, an important library that compiles the background on the twenty-thousand-plus variants that are the probable causes of all disease. The data comes from people who are healthy and those who have diseases, and we use it to try to find the causes of age-related diseases and illnesses. We wanted to know whether centenarians exhibited any of the determinants of diseases, and our theory was that they did not.

We were stunned by what we found. The forty-four centenarians we studied didn't even come close to having perfect genomes. Between them, they had more than 230 variants that ClinVar identified as most likely to cause age-related illnesses, such as Parkinson's disease, Alzheimer's disease, inflammatory diseases (including heart disease), and cancers. They exhibited an average of five to six variants that should have caused disease but didn't. Most striking, two of the centenarians had variants that are a major risk for Alzheimer's (APOE4) — the textbooks say they should have been suffering from dementia at age seventy and dead at eighty — but they were alive and mentally well at one hundred plus! As for the million other variants we looked at, on average, the centenarians had as many variants that are genetically associated with age-related diseases as the control group had.

So with our first hypothesis shot down, we turned to another.

CENTENARIANS' INTERACTIONS WITH THEIR ENVIRONMENTS

A one-hundred-year-old Japanese artist is being interviewed for a newspaper piece about working long after the average retirement age.

"What's the secret of your longevity?" the reporter asks.

The artist finishes cleaning his paintbrush. "I don't know, but I really love fish. I eat it twice a day, and so does my father."

"Your *father*? How old is *he*?"

"He's 125. He eats fish *three* times a day. Would you like to meet him?"

"Sure. Where is he?"

"He's helping my grandfather herd the cattle."

"Your *grandfather*? I suppose he eats fish *four* times a day."

"No, Grandfather *hates* fish."

As with most jokes, there's a lot of truth in this one. Just when you think you've isolated the cause of something, new information complicates the picture. While the discussion of nature versus nurture is ongoing, I was starting to see centenarians' longevity as a cooperative effort between nature and nurture or, more specifically, between genetics and environment. Studies correlating the age at which the parents died and the age at which their children died seemed to suggest that the genetic influence on aging accounts for only about 20 percent of the variations in life span and that environment is responsible for the rest.

But then again, I could see a problem with this low assessment of the genetic contribution in my own family. My grandfather Dov had a heart attack and died at age sixty-eight, while my father, David, had a heart attack at the same age but didn't die till sixteen years later, thanks to bypass surgery. So the relationship of mortality between parents and children changed not because of a difference in aging (they both had heart attacks at the same age) but because of the change in the environment, which in this case was medical intervention. Meanwhile, studies of identical twins who were separated early in life and had different levels of health and different diseases in midlife suggest that genetics account for about 25 percent of the variations in life span. That means that even if you have genes that increase your risk for type 2 diabetes, if you're physically active, eat healthy foods, and manage your stress, you may never develop the disease. So the effects of genes and the effects of environment are not easy to isolate, but as we learn more about genetics' share of the responsibility, we can plan better strategies to protect ourselves from the environment.

All that said, though, all bets are off when it comes to people with exceptional longevity. Other studies suggest that for people with such long life spans, genetics may deserve up to 80 percent of the credit. We still had questions about how much environment might have added to our SuperAgers' longevity, though, so we began a study to assess their lifestyle factors.

The study included 477 Ashkenazi Jews who had been living independently as of ages 95–109. Our nurse, Bill Grainer, collected data on body measurements and administered study questionnaires to gather information on lifestyle factors. In addition to asking them about their habits, we asked them why they thought they lived so long, and all in all, their responses were not what I was expecting. Here are the top ten reasons they gave us:

#10: Helping Those in Need

Many of our 477 SuperAgers volunteered and worked in service of others throughout their lives, even past the century mark. At age ninety-five, Fanny Freund serves as a vital link between the generations as a volunteer for the Dorot Foundation, which creates mutually beneficial relationships between seniors and younger people. During visits facilitated by the foundation, she hosts students at her home for discussions of her family's experiences during the Holocaust and her time on a kibbutz in Israel. Another SuperAger, 104-year-old Lilly (Brock) Port, wrote *Access: The Guide to a Better Life for Disabled Americans* (Yonkers, NY: Consumers Union, 1978), one of the first books to empower the disabled with economic information specific to their situation, during her time as director of consumer education at the Department of Consumer Affairs. She also provided education by way of a consumer affairs radio show. And Irving Kahn served as a trustee emeritus for the Jewish Foundation for Education of Women and founded the New York City Job and Career Center, which helped prepare high school students for the workforce.

#9: Belief in God or Spirituality

I assumed that a good many of our Super-Agers would mention God or spirituality as a reason for healthy longevity, because when we ask them how they feel, they often say something like, "I'm feeling good, thank God." But only 6 percent included spirituality among their reasons for longevity. That said, though, a significant number of our SuperAgers still keep the faith. Fanny is among those who regularly attend synagogue and remain active in their spiritual practice. She says that when her husband of sixty-three years was alive, the synagogue kept them so busy at their separate duties and activities that they rarely saw each other except nights and weekends.

#8: Luck

We weren't surprised that luck made a showing on the list, but we *were* surprised that it placed so highly. Even at age ninety-seven, chemist Morton Rosoff — a *scientist* — largely credits luck for his longevity. And that's coming from a SuperAger who's been defying the odds from the start. Six weeks after Morton was born, he came down with pneumonia and doctors didn't expect him to survive, but he recovered, and in the nine-plus decades since, he's also recovered from heart bypass surgery and a pulmonary embolism that involved such a large blood clot that, again, doctors considered him a lost cause. Though he acknowledges that it's "not very Einsteinian," he seems to speak for many of our SuperAgers when he says he thinks life span is largely a matter of chance. But Morton also happens to have an older sister, one-hundred-year-old Dorothy, so he may have more than luck on his side.

#7: Keeping Busy and Active

Forty-seven percent of men and 43 percent of women said staying busy was a reason for their longevity. And for some, working was part of the equation; 20 percent of the men and 8 percent of the women said they thought it played a role. The life of Harold Laufman may be the strongest argument for the "staying busy" hypothesis. Harold, who died at age ninety-eight, was a modern-day Renaissance man who packed his "extra years" with *doing*. When I asked him to list his interests for me, the list he came up with was a very short one: "Everything." Besides his career as a surgeon, he was an accomplished illustrator and painter, and in his eighth decade of life, he began a career in bioengineering. For the next twenty years, he approached life the same way he had for much of his first seventy — by balancing career with all his other passions and doing his best to explore "everything."

The subject of engagement with life was a favorite topic of discussion whenever I saw Harold: Was his level of engagement the reason for his longevity, or did "good genes" simply make it possible for Harold to thrive for all those years? Whatever the answer, Harold and many other SuperAgers make a convincing case for the benefits of making the absolute most of every day.

6: Not Smoking and Moderate Drinking
Only about 40 percent of the men and 60 percent of the women said they avoided smoking and believed that this contributed

to their longevity. Like his older sister Helen, Irving was a longtime smoker, not kicking the habit until he was about fifty, when he quit to set an example for his children. And many of the SuperAgers who did not smoke had spouses who did, but the secondhand smoke did not appear to have negative consequences for them. Morton's wife, Anne, for example, was a smoker throughout their fifty-four-year marriage, adding to the considerable odds against his exceptional longevity. But those decades of being exposed to secondhand smoke have not taken a detectable toll on Morton.

As for alcohol consumption, we don't know how much protection the SuperAgers have against its effects, because only 24 percent of the men and 12 percent of the women reported drinking alcohol daily.

#5: Social or Family Support

The fact that SuperAgers' fifth most common reason for exceptional longevity was social or family support didn't surprise us, because all the people in our study reported having layers of supportive family members in addition to outside help from social service agencies and in-home aides. Evelyn Edelstein, for example, says she's blessed with three attentive sons, five grandchildren, and two great-grandchildren, and at age ninety-nine, she had the opportunity to see her granddaughter graduate from Yale. She also has friends who range in age from the seventies to early nineties, and she sees all of them often. Meanwhile, in addition to her synagogue family, Fanny sees her sons and their families regularly, and judging by the lift in her voice, FaceTiming with her grandchildren and seven-year-old great-grandson — "a lovely little guy" named Lev — is her greatest joy. "Oh my God, that's the best — I love FaceTime — because he's so cute."

As important as family and friends are to our SuperAgers, it's possible that it wasn't ranked higher because most of the people in our study have lost the most influential partner of their life and their best friends.

#4: Positive Attitude

After enduring significant hardships early in life, my wife's grandmother Frieda emerged from it all with an unshakable optimism, and that kind of positive outlook is a hallmark of many of our SuperAgers. After her family moved to the Bronx from Poland when she was sixteen, she spent the next forty years living close to the poverty line like many immigrants, but she ultimately prevailed, living to age 102 and finding joy all along the way. "No matter the difficulty that one encountered, she always gave you the belief that it'll get better soon," her son (and my father-in-law) Jerry Rubenstein says.

Irma Daniel, who also moved to America from Europe with her family, demonstrated the same kind of emotional resilience. Having fled Germany in response to the attacks on Jews initiated by Adolf Hitler, her family greeted the challenge of starting their lives over with gratitude and optimism. "This was, for us, a fantastic beginning," she told me with the smile that never seemed to leave her face. Even in her eleventh decade of life — she died at 106 — she was grateful for the quality of life she enjoyed. "I think it's wonderful to get that old and have all your faculties," she said. In our study, 19 percent of the SuperAgers said they think this positive way of seeing the world and their lives is a reason for their longevity.

#3: Physical Activity

Considering that four-star nutrition isn't common among our SuperAger study participants (see #2), I thought that maybe they were exercising enough to make up the difference, but only 20 percent of them (more men than women) believed that physical activity played a role in their life span. And even though physical activity was the third most common answer they gave to explain their extended life spans, their histories showed that not many of them were especially active. Frieda was a perfect case in point. "She didn't believe in exercise," Jerry says, but she lived to age 102 anyway, the same age at which her father died.

There are exceptions, of course — like Jerry, who's part of our study because he is the offspring of a centenarian. At age eighty-nine, he still plays two sets of singles tennis a day and appears to be in great health. And Lilly, who makes it a practice to walk up and down the stairs of her home sixty-five times a day. Speaking of steps, she also climbed the three-thousand-plus steps at Machu Picchu during a recent visit. And she's a regular at her gym, where she is often found walking a treadmill, riding a stationary bike, working with weights, or taking a tai chi class. "You have to be active — exercise and walking, lots of walking," she says when asked for some tips for living a long, healthy life. "And skiing and bicycle riding and . . ." And the list goes on.

2: Diet

This response surprised me because the SuperAgers' diets frequently included fatty meats, schmaltz (rendered chicken fat), and sweets. In fact, the only complaint I ever got about the trained nurse who administered the questionnaires was that he didn't accept the high-fat baked goods that the SuperAgers had made for their meetings. I would get phone calls saying, "He was a very nice man, but why wouldn't he eat a piece of my cake?" Once I explained to him that he needed to accept all edible gifts and that he was free to give them away to the first takers he ran into, I got no more complaints.

But whatever the larger truth is, we certainly have our share of SuperAgers like Lilly, who take diet very seriously. "I am not letting myself eat as much as I would like to, and I'm trying to stay away from fattening things," she says. And for her, it's been a lifelong habit, not just something she got smart about in her later years. At sixteen, she decided that she had put on too much weight, so she cut out the cookies and lost thirty pounds. And judging by photos taken throughout her life, she consistently kept them off.

#1: Good Genes

Despite all the external factors that might figure into longevity — the factors that the SuperAgers have control over and often *do* take control over — they believe that genes are the biggest determinant of life span. And of course, I agree. Remember that exceptional longevity tends to run in families, and that's a strong indicator that environment and lifestyle can carry most of us only so far. In chapter 2, we will explore some striking genetic similarities among people with exceptional longevity.

DO AS I SAY, NOT AS I DO

Once we knew what centenarians thought was keeping them alive, we were able to look at how their opinions compared with their lab results and health histories. And yes, we were surprised again. The results of the lifestyle factor tests made it clear that it wasn't healthy habits keeping the SuperAgers alive and well. Even though many of them gave credit to their diets and physical activity for their extended years, most of them weren't living these beliefs at the time of the study, nor had they lived them during their early years. Based on the National Health and Nutrition Examination Survey (NHANES-I), they had mean body mass indexes (BMI) similar to the national average, but almost half of them had been overweight or even obese for most of their lives. Sixty percent of men and 30 percent of women had been heavy smokers for more than thirty-five years, and 20 percent drank alcohol daily for much of their lives. And fewer than half of them had been physically active over the course of their lifetimes — only 43 percent of the men and 47 percent of the women. The numbers for restricting calories were even lower: 21 percent of the men and 27 percent of the women. While plant-based diets are often credited with greater health and longevity, fewer than 3 percent of the SuperAgers in our study were vegetarians.

So much for healthy lifestyles getting credit for long lives! We were astonished that our study subjects had habits that were as bad as or worse than the habits of those in the control group. It was clear that as a group, people with exceptional longevity do not have healthier practices or habits than the general population. When we completed this study, the important takeaway for us was that our third hypothesis appeared to be correct — the SuperAgers were somehow being protected by genetic differences that the general population doesn't have. But when the results of the study were published in 2010, the media put an inaccurate spin on the story, and so did many people who saw me interviewed for a network news segment.

Shortly after the interview, I was at a coffee shop when I was stopped by a middle-aged man who recognized me from the interview. "You changed my life," he said. "I saw your interview when I was at the gym. My grandmother is one hundred years old, so I don't need to exercise anymore."

It got worse. Jay Leno, then host of *The Tonight Show,* said, "Scientists at the Albert Einstein College of Medicine — I don't know where that is — showed that the secret for successful longevity is eating, drinking, and not exercising . . . And the good thing about it is that if you die anyway, you don't care."

Of course, our findings applied only to centenarians, and I made sure that I said that in every interview I gave, but people didn't want to hear that part. Even for people who inherit longevity genes, I recommend a healthy diet and regular physical activity. What was ironic was that the media had a field day with this study and all but ignored the most significant discoveries we were making. The real news was our realization that something must be protecting the centenarians, some undiscovered genetic alteration that helps, not hurts. Something that keeps these wildly different individuals living longer and far better than the rest of us. We have already identified some of these defenses, and research aimed at using them in treatments is under way. (I'll explain these in detail in chapter 2.) When we made this discovery about centenarians' remarkable genetic makeup, it was the first key to unlocking how we age and how we can age later and better. By that point, the study had been under way for five years, and this was our first big win.

Two:
Why We Age

At his annual checkup, a
ninety-two-year-old man said,
"Doctor, do you think I'll make it
to a hundred? I don't drink, smoke,
eat rich food, or have a lot of sex."

His doctor asked, "So why do you want to
live to be a hundred?"

Studying the biology of longevity and aging
has led to some surprising and promising
insights about how and why we age and,
more important, how we can age later and
slower. With each new discovery geroscientists make, we get closer to creating a future
in which the golden years are truly golden.
As a physician with a background in molecular genetics and endocrinology, I am well
versed in the medical problems that plague
the elderly, but until I met my wife's grandmother Frieda, I had never deeply ques-

74

tioned the biology of longevity. Her vitality as she grew older was in such stark contrast with people twenty years younger, so I couldn't help wondering: Just what *is* aging?

We know that our bodies, organs, and even our cells experience wear and tear, consistent with a law of physics — the second law of thermodynamics. Like appliances, all these physical objects break down over time. We also know that environmental factors like what we eat and drink, whether we exercise or smoke, and how well we sleep may slow or accelerate aging. So we have a variety of interesting theories about the root causes. One of the more controversial theories suggests that aging is programmed — that our cells receive biological signals that tell them when to deteriorate and when to die. At an event on aging at Gordon Research Conferences, I led a panel discussion about whether this is true — whether our bodies are programmed to age and, if so, whether they can be *un*programmed. Even colleagues who are typically provocateurs were subdued, with few wanting to defend the notion that the indignities of aging are inevitable. One scientist, Hong Gil Nam from South Korea, presented illuminating data showing how tree leaves are programmed to age, not because of wear and tear or external environmental factors but because the tree itself sends out a signal telling the leaves to change color, die, and drop from the branch. I can still remember the silence that blanketed the room after he delivered his conclusions. What did this mean for humans? Are we programmed to decay, too? The implications were unsettling. But as I gave it more thought, I realized that the leaves are programmed to die, but the tree *itself* is not, and neither are we. Although our cells can activate in response to stress and aging by way of a program to die, known as *apoptosis,* or stop dividing, if they are damaged and cannot be repaired, that does not directly program our death.

Jan Vijg at Einstein conducted a study with Vera Gorbunova, University of Rochester; Laura Niedernhofer and Paul Robbins, University of Minnesota; and others that showed that in many species, as we age, more of our cells develop mutations. Genomic instability — a high frequency of mutations — is one of the hallmarks of aging, and this team showed that mutations accumulate in part because repair mechanisms are increasingly impaired. If repair is impaired, cells can die or stop dividing, leading to a decrease in the sizes of organs. And if the repair mechanisms fail, cells can become cancerous.

At least part of the problem lies in the mitochondria, whose number and function decline with age. As the mitochondria suffer free radical damage and accumulate damage in their own DNA — which is commonly believed to be the primary culprit in the decline — their energy production may become impaired and cause apoptosis. Mitochondrial dysfunction is associated with many health risks, including heart, kidney, liver, and gastrointestinal diseases. Decline in mitochondrial numbers and function is also implicated in declines in vision, hearing, and skin condition. And impaired mitochondrial function is associated with major metabolic conditions, such as obesity and diabetes.

In our initial studies with Ashkenazi Jews, we did not find any differences between centenarians' mitochondria subtypes and control groups' mitochondria subtypes, but Joseph Attardi, California Institute of Technology, had previously observed a mitochondrial mutation that occurs much more frequently in Italian centenarians than in the rest of the Italian population. This prompted us to analyze our own population more deeply, and while we could not confirm the genetic finding from Italian centenarians, we *did* find an aging-related increase in the incidence of another mutation that was not inherited and occurred by chance during early development. This finding alerted us to a new biology of aging related to the mitochondria, which we'll cover in chapter 5.

Evolution has faced a lot of challenges and perfected our biology through trial-and-error experiments over billions of years. So when scientists make a discovery, we first ask, "Why did evolution create it this way?" Evolution prioritizes reproduction, so that may be why the aging process picks up speed *after* reproduction. While it's true that men can reproduce well into their seventies and beyond, the majority of men fathering babies are in their twenties. Once we've passed our DNA to our children, there's nothing else we can do to contribute to the evolution of our ability to age no matter how long we live. However, there's a really interesting hypothesis about that. Based on a combination of biology and sociology, the "grandparent hypothesis" suggests that orphans (whose parents generally weren't resilient enough to withstand the aging process and died relatively young) don't do as well as people who grew up with parents and grandparents. The grandparents who had survived were biologically resilient, and because of that, they had time to accumulate wealth and wisdom and have more children and grandchildren. So in evolutionary terms, the DNA that allowed the grandparents to age better had the effects of populating and strengthening the biology for the next generations. That's one example of the many aging theories out there that are correct, but it's important to remember that there's much more to the story.

One of my favorite explanations for aging is the *antagonistic pleiotropy theory,* which suggests that biological resources we need for reproduction when we're young may end up hurting us when we're old. In 1957, George C. Williams offered this hypothesis that rapid aging is the price paid to achieve better reproduction. For example, we need cholesterol to build the membrane of cells, including those associated with reproduction, so it's possible that people who have high cholesterol levels are going to have more reproductive success. But after their children are born, this cholesterol can eventually turn against them, harm their blood vessels, and increase their risk of heart diseases and stroke. On the other hand, we need cholesterol throughout our lives to build cell membranes and for healthy brain function. But scientists have found that nature provides many examples of exchanges between longevity and reproduction that support this theory. In numerous research studies conducted with a variety of animals, the animals that reproduced did not live as long as those that were prevented from reproducing. And the animals with the most offspring died first. So it looks like there is an exchange between reproduction and longevity, but the evidence is far from conclusive. For instance, there are studies showing that increasing reproduction in fruit flies *extends* their life span.

GENOTYPE

A genotype is a change in the sequence of a gene (also known as a variant or SNP). It is important if it is linked to a single trait like red hair, or a disease like diabetes.

When we began our Longevity Genes Project, we were still curious about the exchange between reproduction and longevity. I jokingly proposed that maybe for humans, it's more about raising kids than birthing them. Research conducted by Alan Shuldiner, endocrinologist, geneticist, and vice president of Regeneron Pharmaceuticals, has shown that the more offspring that Amish parents have (up to thirteen), the longer the parents live. A friend and colleague, Alan has conducted genetic studies with the Amish because they have only two hundred to three hundred founders. It's likely that there's a social explanation for the results, considering that in such a society the more kids you have, the more kids are available to take care of you as you age.

In our medical history survey, we ask the offspring of the centenarians and the members of the control group how many children their parents had and found that, besides having them later in life than their peers who lived to an average life expectancy, the centenarians had significantly fewer children — both the men and the women in our study had on average from one-half to one fewer child than the average. And since the centenarians — who have longevity genotypes — have fewer offspring, the number of people who possess a longevity genotype may have decreased with every generation. While income, education, and other factors affect birth rate, the centenarians in our study are more alike than different when it comes to education and income levels. They also did not have access to very effective birth control methods, so there seems to be a lot of evolutionary pressure to eliminate longevity genes. With this in mind, it's possible that the ages of Abraham — 175 — and Moses — 120 — recorded in the Old Testament and the Torah were true. Not to mention Methuselah, who's said to have lived to 964, and Noah, said to have reached 960. Maybe we're losing longevity genes because of a low rate of reproduction among those with exceptional longevity (Abraham had only two sons, one delivered when he was one hundred years old).

We also wanted to see if there was any correlation between longevity in women and the age of menopause. As I looked through the stack of completed surveys on my desk, I noticed that nearly all the female centenarians had begun menopause exactly at age fifty. *Wow, this is impossible,* I thought. And there were too many cases to be a coincidence, so I called our nurse, Bill, who had administered the surveys, to ask if he had any insight into why so many of the women started menopause when they were exactly fifty.

"Well, I ask them when they stopped having their menses, and most of them don't remember," he said. "So I say, 'Fifty?' And they say, 'Yes, fifty.' "

We had a good laugh about that, but it's a perfect example of why research survey questions are standardized and need to be asked a certain way, which we eventually did once we homed in on the questions that were most important for us to ask.

RECENT THEORIES

When I tell people that I study centenarians, one of the questions I get is: "If I want to live to one hundred, should I move to a blue zone?" *Blue zones* are the places with the world's longest-living populations, as identified by *National Geographic* fellow Dan Buettner. He found these populations in Loma Linda, California; Ikaria, Greece; Okinawa, Japan; Nicoya, Costa Rica; and Sardinia, Italy, and he looked for commonalities among the people there to see what lifestyles and backgrounds contributed to the longest lives. These locations don't all have more centenarians on average than other places, but the people who live there stay healthy for longer and live longer on average than people in other locations.

Buettner found nine common denomina-

83

tors among the people in the blue zones:

1. They make moderate physical activity part of every day.
2. They identify a life purpose.
3. They practice sacred daily rituals that may manage stress.
4. They consume a moderate number of calories each day.
5. They eat relatively large amounts of vegetables, greens, tubers, beans, and nuts.
6. They consume alcohol moderately or don't drink at all.
7. They engage in spiritual or religious practice.
8. They enjoy active, integrated family lives.
9. They have close, devoted friends and regularly participate in supportive social communities.

All these common denominators can contribute to a longer health span and life span, but I think the most significant common denominator is genetics. For example, in Sardinia, there are three villages that are very close to each other that have a population of one-hundred-year-old males. But there are many other small villages nearby that have the same environment — the same climate, trees, and pretty much everything else — that don't have populations that live longer than others on average.

The same situation exists on Ikaria. There are more centenarians on the island per capita than on nearby islands, which have the same climate, plants, and animals. So while blue zones may show an interaction between genes and environment, unless the genetics of these populations are studied, we can't know whether it's the environment, the genes, or the interaction of the genes with the environment that's responsible for the longevity. I think the blue zones are great, and there's good reason to believe that living in a blue zone may help to increase health span and life span. But no matter where centenarians live, they are usually genetically unique, and we need to keep in mind that not everyone who lives in a blue zone makes it to a hundred years old.

So the jury is still out on the major underlying factors that contribute to blue zones, but they're not the only hot longevity topic to make the news. Dr. Elizabeth H. Blackburn, who co-authored *The Telomere Effect* with Dr. Elissa Epel, was awarded a Nobel Prize for discovering the molecular nature of telomeres, which are DNA extensions at the ends of chromosomes that carry no genetic information but keep the chromosomes compact and protected, like the tips of shoelaces, and for codiscovering the enzyme called *telomerase.* As we age, telomeres become shorter, and Blackburn and others promoted the hypothesis that this shortening drives aging. In our studies at Einstein, we'd found that centenarians had longer telomeres than people who were eighty-five years old, and the centenarians' offspring also had longer telomeres than their control groups.

Blackburn often mentioned our high-profile study because it showed some alterations in the genes of telomerase, although we did not know their functional importance. That seemed to support the theory that the longer our telomeres are, the longer we live. But we need to do long-term studies to better understand this conclusion, because we don't know if the people who had longer-than-average telomeres at age eighty-five started out with longer ones or if they became shorter more slowly than other people's. Maybe our centenarians started out with telomeres of the same length as the average person's but they didn't lose as much length over their lifetimes. Or maybe their telomeres were much longer than average when they were born. With more research, I think we'll find that when people age more slowly, the length of their telomeres is longer because they started with longer telomeres at birth or had less telomere "attrition." So while having long telomeres may predict good health that doesn't mean they cause longevity.

In a lab next to mine at Einstein, Dr. Ron DePinho studied mice in which telomeres are made shorter by knocking out the telomerase enzyme — the enzyme that elongates telomeres — and the first generation of these mice did not age more than those that were not manipulated. On the other hand, lengthening telomeres by telomerase over-expression will usually cause cancer. Blackburn carefully measured average telomere length in the blood of thousands of people and showed that those with the shortest telomeres were at risk for heart disease and those with the longest telomeres were at risk for cancer. Interestingly, mice have much longer telomeres than humans, and Ron argues that his mice did not get old because their shortest telomeres were longer than humans'. When telomeres are manipulated to become shorter over generations, the mice do age more quickly. However, the problem with this argument is that while mice age in ways similar to humans, they do it in a much shorter time period and die at around three years of age with longer telomeres, suggesting that telomeres are really not a major factor in aging for animals or humans.

So it seems that even though the health of centenarians and their offspring is characterized by longer telomeres, having average telomere length is optimal for most of us. Also, telomere length can be rapidly regulated by stress, which shortens them, and prayers, which lengthen them, suggesting flexibility in their length even if they become shorter on average. So measuring the length has no predictive value.

One of the latest theories of aging — and my favorite — is presented by my friend and colleague David Sinclair in *Lifespan: Why We Age — and Why We Don't Have To.* The information theory of aging proposes that we age and become more susceptible to diseases because our cells lose information. DNA stores information digitally, but the cells have an analog format that can modulate the function of genes in the sequence of the DNA. The analogy David uses to explain this theory is that of a CD player (or, for us older folks, a record player). The digital information is the "song," and the scratches on the surface of the disc represent the accumulated effects of aging in the DNA. Another way to think of it is that the DNA, including longevity genes, is the hardware and epigenetics is the software. And the question we're asking is how to remove the scratches. We can find the mechanisms of aging through observing and experimenting with the changes in the digital information. The analog information is changing all the time because of our interaction with the environment. It's the epigenetic information that tells a cell whether it's a liver cell or a hair cell. When we grow old, cells become confused because epigenetic mechanisms are scrambling the information. That's why fat cells start showing up in the liver and hair cells develop instead of skin cells. The last example is why older people often have hair sprouting from their ears and other places where it didn't used to grow.

Methylation is an epigenetic process — specifically a chemical reaction between DNA and a unit of organic compounds known as a *methyl group* — that can either activate or deactivate genes. Each of the body's cells have exactly the same chromosomes, but we don't need to use every one of the genes in every cell. Methylation helps to decide what type of cell is formed, such as a fat cell, a liver cell, or a cell for another specific part of the body.

THE SEARCH FOR PROTECTION FROM AGING

Currently at Einstein, Gil Atzmon, my first postdoc fellow in genetics and now the core director of the longevity projects, is looking at epigenetic methylation in the stem cells of our families of centenarians. The methylation patterns in centenarians' stem cells are dramatically different from those of the control group, and those of centenarians' offspring are different from those of the age-matched control group. Since methylation occurs across the genome in millions of locations, this work is expensive, and its analysis is ongoing.

Meanwhile, hundreds of researchers worldwide are measuring proteins and metabolites, including hormone levels, to discover biomarkers that change as we age. We are finding that the changes in some of these measurements don't do harm — they don't seem to drive aging — while the changes in others *may* cause aging. What's harder to decipher is which changes are responsible for the breakdown that occurs with aging, which ones are protecting us, and which ones do both. And it's critical that we figure this out — if we mistakenly change something that's protective, we make more trouble. Some mechanisms such as inflammation, which becomes more common with age, can be protective or destructive under different circumstances. We know that inflammation can contribute to chronic disease, so it might seem that we should find a way to stop it entirely, but we need inflammation to help us fight infection. Without it, we'd die.

Inflammaging, a term coined by immunologist Claudio Franceschi, reflects biological measures of inflammatory factors that are expressed in the elderly mainly by musculoskeletal pain that most of them suffer from. Some of the inflammation is caused by cells that stop dividing but do not die. These senescent cells — a.k.a. "zombie" cells — accumulate with age and can go rogue and secrete inflammatory factors and other proteins known as SASP (senescence associating secretory proteins) that may change their local environment and cause cancer.

We are also learning that some mechanisms, including sex hormones and growth hormones, fade as we age to protect us, and replacing or supplementing them has not proved to increase health span or life span. Estrogen and testosterone are prime examples of hormones that decline with age, and as an endocrinologist, I used to think that a lot of aging had to do with this decline and that hormonal treatment might slow aging. But this theory has proved to be largely erroneous. I believe evolution has a good reason for menopause. Tom Kirkwood, a scientist, colleague, and friend, argued in a provocative paper that if reproduction did not have an age cutoff in humans, many mothers would die relatively young because childbirth becomes riskier with age, and in many cases, mothers and grandmothers would therefore be unavailable to support the younger offspring. Many animals do not go into menopause, so this effect might be explained as a "side effect" of humans' evolving to stand and walk on two feet instead of hands and feet. This position led to a narrowing of the pelvis, which had been wider when weight was distributed over four limbs rather than two. With more available nutrition, the babies also became bigger, and in combination with the erect position, this made large babies difficult to deliver and could have claimed the lives of many mothers. While a number of factors contribute to the rise in Cesarean sections in the past decades, one of the factors is overnutrition in pregnant women relative to their pelvis size.

Since we always need to consider the reasons that evolution planned our biology as it is, it's usually best to proceed with caution when we attempt to alter those plans. For example, while hormone replacement therapy was all the rage for decades, a long-term national study conducted by the Women's Health Initiative (WHI) found that many effects of estrogen were harmful in some postmenopausal women. In the study, which involved women who were an average age of sixty, the women who were given estrogen had more clusters of age-related diseases — such as heart attacks, more breast cancer, and more cognitive decline — than women in the same age range who were given a placebo. So while women who received estrogen did prefer not to have hot flashes, sleep disturbances, and other distressing symptoms of menopause and liked some of the positive effects, such as improvements in their skin and prevention of colon cancer, the estrogen replacement was harmful in terms of protecting against some major age-related diseases. Since the publication of this study, other studies have reported a decrease of up to 25 percent in the incidence of breast cancer in the United States.

Declining estrogen and resultant menopause appear to be protective against aging, and if that's true, averting these conditions is the wrong thing to do. By the way, the same goes for declining testosterone in men — replacement therapies among men with very low testosterone improve some symptoms but increase the risks for other conditions. In fact, the risk-to-benefit ratio led doctors to stop recommending it even to men who are highly deficient in testosterone.

People who had been staunch believers in hormone replacement therapy were shocked by the results of the WHI study and are looking for windows of opportunity where the treatments will have the desired effects without doing harm. There are studies that suggest there may be a time frame between ages fifty and sixty when hormone replacement therapy could be beneficial, but as I explained earlier, estrogen appears to be a hormone that is beneficial in young women but harmful in older women, so we still have a lot to learn. And since people biologically age at different rates, we would need to pinpoint the right time frame for each person. Beyond that, even if we can provide the therapy during the optimal period, the benefits may end shortly after that time frame ends.

The WHI was a billion-dollar study that was controversial from the start. Many scientists and clinicians asked why it was necessary to spend so much money on a clinical study when there was already strong evidence from association studies. They had concluded from those studies that there was evidence that although estrogen carries a risk of thrombosis and strokes for some women, it does many good things for post-menopausal women, chief among them clearing the symptoms of menopause — hot flashes, sleep disturbances, mood changes, and vaginal dryness. Some animal models — most of them mice or rats that were supplemented with estrogen or a placebo after having had their ovaries removed at a young age — supported the notion that estrogen has positive effects. (Studies involving *old* mice and rats, whose health usually declined after being treated with estrogen, were largely ignored based on the argument that they were already too old or sick by then.) But the problem with association studies is that they do not account for the varying behaviors and habits of the participants. While many of the women who had been taking estrogen saw improvements, it was because they were taking very good care of themselves in other ways, not because they were receiving estrogen. Many women on estrogen were exercising regularly, did not smoke, took vitamins and supplements, carried less excess weight, and had healthier lifestyles in general than the women who were not taking estrogen. Admittedly, they also took estrogen very early on, rather than starting to take it in their sixties, and that may make a difference.

The WHI, on the other hand, was a clinical study (i.e., some patients received placebos), and it was also double-blind, meaning that neither the doctor nor the patient knew their assignment. And this kind of controlled study is the *only* kind of study that can specifically determine whether a drug works. In the case of estrogen, there's no doubt that it has a youthful effect on a young body, but the question was, can it restore youthfulness to an old body? And the answer is no — an answer that had to come from a double-blind clinical study.

EATING LESS MAY LEAD TO MORE HEALTHY YEARS

When I began studying the science of aging, the theory of cutting calories to increase longevity was being tested in research labs around the globe. Eating less than what we'd normally eat is called *caloric restriction,* and in animals, it turned out to have one of the most reproducible effects on slowing aging, increasing average and maximal life span, and increasing health span. For years, caloric restriction consumed geroscience because it was the only reliable method we'd found that could significantly extend longevity and delay the occurrence of age-related diseases.

In an experiment that is easily replicated in many rodent species, we restricted rats' calories by 40 percent, and they lived about 40 percent longer than rats that were fed ad libitum — in other words, as much as they wanted. This was very exciting, so labs across the world began looking at why caloric restriction was increasing maximal life span. Collectively, we discovered that caloric restriction reduces age-related pathology, cancers, and other age-related diseases in rodents and slows down most physiological functions. So it not only increases life span but also increases health span. Still more exciting, there was good reason to believe that there would be similar effects in humans. But as a doctor with a specialty in treating type 2 diabetes, I know how difficult it is for people to cut calories. I tell all my patients to lose weight, but less than 3 percent of them are able to do it. If caloric restriction is as effective for people as it is for rats, we will need to isolate the mechanism that makes restriction beneficial and develop drugs or other treatments that

don't involve cutting so many calories —
calorie restriction mimetics. No matter how
hard they try, most people will not be able
to consistently cut calories by 40 percent by
eating less than they normally would at each
meal. For those who manage to do it, we
always say, "I don't know if they'll live
longer, but it will probably feel that way."

UNLOCKING THE SECRETS IN FAT
While our research certainly made it look
like restricting calories was directly related
to less disease and longer lives, I wasn't
convinced that it was the restriction itself
that was producing these dramatic results.
Initially, I thought that eating less prevents
not aging itself but obesity and that the lack
of obesity triggers the protective mechanisms that delay the onset of disease and
extend life. My line of thinking was that rats
that live outdoors run many miles a day to
look for food, so they use a lot of calories. If
we put them in a cage where they can eat as
much as they want — and certainly more
than they would if they lived outdoors —
but can't run around, the experiment is in
some part about obesity versus leanness,
not necessarily about eating a weight-
maintaining diet versus caloric restriction.
It was time to look at fat from a new

perspective, so we set up a study to do just that.

PEPTIDE OR PROTEIN?

Peptides and proteins are both sequences of amino acids, but peptides are smaller. They are generally defined as molecules that consist of up to fifty amino acids, while proteins consist of more than fifty amino acids. Peptides also tend to be less well defined in structure than proteins, which can be organized into complex arrangements.

We used to think that fat tissue was just storage of excess fat, but we've discovered that fat — a.k.a. adipose tissue — has a biology and secretes several hormones and peptides. One of the hormones, called *leptin,* tells the brain when the body has had enough to eat, and years back, many researchers thought that leptin would become a treatment for weight loss. But while it's true that the more fat tissue we have, the more leptin we have, our brain receptors stop responding past a certain point, becoming resistant to the effect of this hormone.

Instead of receiving a signal telling us that we have had enough to eat, the signal is blocked and we feel like we *haven't* had enough. In our own leptin experiments involving rats, we could not elicit in old animals the same effects we elicited in young animals. While caloric restriction generally seemed to reverse aging, even calorically restricted old animals did not respond to leptin. So advanced age seems to be a leptin-resistant state, and we lost interest in leptin as a potential gerotherapeutic supplement that would mimic caloric restriction's effects.

With another hormone, adiponectin, the opposite happens. The more adipose tissue we have, the less adiponectin we have. But considering that this hormone is generally good for all aspects of our metabolism, lowers insulin resistance and inflammation, and has a number of other positive properties, this is not a case where less is more. In our Longevity Genes Project, we had found that centenarians have high adiponectin even though they are not restricting calories. Instead, some of them have a helpful mutation in the adiponectin gene that keeps their levels of this good hormone high and acts as a protective mechanism. For those of us without the beneficial mutation, a little bit of fat works in our favor, but having too much intra-abdominal fat (visceral fat) is at the core of the metabolic decline that occurs with age. Abdominal obesity — think older people who are thin but have big bellies — is the marker for the onset of diseases. This is accepted now, but when I first introduced to the field of gerontology the idea that the biology of adipose tissue might be the mechanism underlying the apparent success of caloric restriction, my theory was viciously attacked.

Being a researcher requires thick skin and an open mind. Things are not always what they appear to be, and when I'm tempted to jump to a conclusion, I recall a story I heard about a photograph that was taken of Pope John Paul II at the wheel of a limousine. As the story goes, the pope had given a sermon at a cathedral in Yonkers, New York, in the mid-'90s, and afterward, a Cadillac limousine was waiting to take him to the airport. When the pope saw his driver, he said, "My son, when I was in Poland, I drove all the time. I really want to drive a Cadillac."

So the driver, not knowing how to say no to the pope, got into the back seat, and the pope headed for JFK. On the way there, he was pulled over for speeding, and the officer asked to see his driver's license.

"I'm sorry, son, I don't have a license," the pope said. "But we're only going a short distance to the airport, so I'm sure we'll be fine."

Not sure what to do, the officer called his captain. "I stopped a limo for speeding, and it's somebody really important," he said.

"Who is it?"

"I don't know."

"You're telling me it's somebody really important, but you don't know who?"

"Well," the officer said, "it *has* to be somebody really important because the pope is his driver."

Had the officer peered into the back seat and seen the driver in his chauffeur uniform, he would have reached a different conclusion. What's obvious is often misleading, so researchers make a habit of peering into the back seat. This is what we had in mind when we constructed a major study to test my theory that the "success" of caloric restriction was actually due to having only a small amount of visceral fat. We could have chalked that success up to caloric restriction, but we decided to look into the back seat by performing a new experiment.

We started with four groups of rats — one group of young rats and three groups of old rats. Of the three groups of old rats, we restricted the calories of one group and let the other groups eat as much as they wanted. By the end of the experiment, the old rats with restricted calories weighed the same amount as the young rats, but the two groups of old rats that ate as much as they wanted were obese, weighing two hundred grams more than the rats in the other groups.

Then we did something dramatic with the two groups of obese rats that required extensive practice and experience. In one group, we performed a surgery where we removed visible deposits of visceral fat from inside the abdomens. In the other group, we removed the same amount of surface (subcutaneous) fat as we'd removed in the form of visceral fat from the other group. In the young group and the older group that had been calorically restricted, we made an incision in their abdominal walls but sutured the wounds without removing fat for the sake of control (known as a sham operation).

We measured all the rats' insulin levels and insulin's action regarding driving glucose out of the bloodstream and into the muscle. One of the hallmarks of the metabolic decline that comes with aging is a decline in sensitivity to the effects of insulin, the hormone we need to store sugar molecules. Insulin is manufactured in the beta cells of the pancreas, and its levels become elevated to overcome the decline in insulin sensitivity. Those of us who can't secrete enough insulin become type 2 diabetics. Obesity accelerates this process because it increases resistance to insulin, so obese people can become diabetic at earlier ages.

The gold standard for determining whole-body insulin sensitivity is the "insulin clamp" test, which my Einstein mentor and colleague Luciano Rosetti and I were the first researchers to apply to rodents and to aging. I had performed insulin clamp studies in humans during medical school at the Technion in Israel, where I worked with my first mentor, Eddy Karnieli, and during fellowships at Yale with leading diabetes researcher Ralph DeFronzo. For the studies, insulin is administered, but glucose concentration is "clamped" so that the study participants' normal blood sugar levels are maintained — they do not go up or down. The more glucose you need to administer to hold glucose levels steady, the more sensitive the body is to insulin. The less glucose you need to administer to maintain the levels, the more resistant the body is to insulin. For the same levels of insulin, much less glucose needs to be administered for elderly people than for young people, because elderly people are generally in an insulin-resistant state. In our studies, when aging animals had their subcutaneous fat removed, they had insulin resistance typical of advanced age. In contrast, old caloric-restricted animals had the same insulin sensitivity as young animals. The group that I was holding my breath about was the group of old rats that had had visceral fat removed. If our theory was correct, their insulin sensitivity would be similar to that of the young and the old caloric-restricted animals, and to our delight, they were. All we had to do to achieve a healthy metabolism in rats that ate as much as they wanted and were also obese was to take out their visceral fat!

We knew we were onto something, and we wanted to see what would happen if we did a similar experiment with a model of diabetic rats. A breed of lab rats known as Zucker fatty rats begins developing diabetes at two months, and by the time they're five months old, 100 percent of them will be diabetic. We removed our rats' visceral fat at two months of age, and by the time they were five months old, only 20 percent of them had diabetes. It looked like a victory until we hit the end of month six, by which time all the rats in the study were diabetic. At first, we were disappointed, but then we realized that the rats' visceral fat had grown back and that that's why they became diabetic. Further study revealed that they would become diabetic when 60 percent of the visceral fat had grown back. As long as they had less than 40 percent, though, they did not become diabetic, so the experiment ended up proving exactly what we had theorized.

But the ultimate study was the one we did with more than 150 rats that were divided into three groups. One group was fed as much as they wanted. The second group had their calories restricted. And the third group ate as much as they wanted, but we removed their visceral fat at the beginning of the experiment. We also performed a sham operation on the first two groups, surgically opening and closing them without removing visceral fat.

The caloric restriction did what we expected it to do, and the restricted group lived about 40 percent longer than the group with no caloric restriction. The group that had had visceral fat removed didn't live quite as long, but they did live about 20 percent longer than the control. So with the visceral fat removed, their maximum life span was close to that of the caloric-restricted animals. What this means is that nutrients themselves, or the time they are administered, are playing a role in aging, but taking out the visceral fat has significant effects on longevity.

While we won't be doing this surgical procedure on people, we may be able to develop a less invasive treatment or drug that does the same thing. I have been helping a company that developed a method to melt intra-abdominal fat that has demonstrated a significant metabolic improvement in monkeys, and now they're starting human trials. So that's good news on the horizon, and I also have some wonderful news about subcutaneous fat. We're learning that having a little bit of fat under the skin is a good thing. Not just because it can act as a protective barrier against viruses, germs, and other substances that manage to penetrate the skin but also because it produces the "good" peptides and fat hormones like adiponectin, which as I mentioned earlier is found at high levels in centenarians.

CALORIC RESTRICTION:
A MIXED BAG OF EFFECTS

Around the same time as our rat study, researchers Richard Weindruch, Joseph Kemnitz, and Rozalyn Anderson at the University of Wisconsin and Donald Ingram, Julie Mattison, and Rafael de Cabo at the National Institute on Aging in Baltimore studied the effects of caloric restriction on primates. The experiments were different, but in both cases, the animals that were permitted to eat as much as they wanted became obese from excess calories and lack of exercise, which is also what happens with people. Both studies showed that a variety of age-related diseases, including diabetes and cardiovascular disease, were delayed in the monkeys with restricted diets. These are the same diseases that are delayed when you fight obesity. But only the University of Wisconsin study showed a significant increase in life span.

At one point, I was one of the reviewers on the Wisconsin program, and when we visited the research facility at the university, I wasn't the only one who noticed that over the past year or so, the animals being fed restricted calories had come to weigh almost as much as those that were permitted to eat as much as they wanted. "There's only one explanation here," I said, "and that is that somebody sabotaged the experiment." The other reviewers agreed, and we wondered what the study's researchers would say about this.

When we arrived for the review panel the next day, one of the researchers explained that a caretaker had felt sorry for the animals with restricted diets and gave them almost as much food as she gave the control group. I didn't want our animal care workers to do the same thing in any of our studies, so when I got back to Einstein, I attended their next meeting and told them what had happened in Wisconsin. I explained that while the concerned caretaker thought she was helping the animals on restricted diets by feeding them more, if they had gotten fewer calories, they would have had healthier and longer lives.

Since caloric restriction looked like it was extending health span and life span, the research community was curious to learn how it affected levels of growth hormones, sex hormones, thyroid hormones, insulin levels, and cortisol levels. As it turned out, animal models whose levels of hormones were maintained at caloric-restricted levels in isolation did not realize extended life spans. So far, the only decrease that's known to make a difference in longevity is the decrease in growth hormones. (More about this in chapter 5.) As for levels of cortisol, which is a stress hormone, they went up because restricting the diet by 40 percent causes stress, but when cortisol is administered to old animals, it actually shortens their life spans.

From my standpoint, the study about caloric restriction that's most relevant to humans is one that showed how genetics change the effects of caloric restriction. Jim Nelson, a colleague from San Antonio, gathered other colleagues to this fascinating study in which he bred two mice that were genetically very different. Eventually, the mice produced male and female offspring with forty-one genetically distinct backgrounds. All the mice were either fed ad libitum or fed restricted diets, but unexpectedly, only about half of the caloric-restricted animals lived longer than the ad libitum mice, and the other half lived shorter. This means that genetic background is very important and that caloric restriction cannot be universally applied. Whether caloric restriction will lead to a longer life in humans also depends on our genetic backgrounds. And how many calories we should restrict ourselves to may also depend on our

DNA. Among other limitations of this study, it's possible that the researchers would have seen more longevity if the calorie restriction had been less severe than 40 percent. If they had cut 20 percent of the mice's calories, I think that significantly more than half of the calorie-restricted mice would have outlived the ad libitum mice.

It's possible that caloric restriction produces the most benefits for the obese and does harm to people who are of average weight or leaner. Yet there are thousands of people who *are not* obese who religiously follow a diet of calorie restriction with optimum nutrition (CRON). These people, popularly referred to as CRONies, eat a low-protein, low-fat, high-plant diet and consume only about nineteen hundred calories a day. I once gave a talk about caloric restriction and adipose tissues at the University of Cambridge, and during the luncheon that followed, I found myself surrounded by a group of CRONies. I recognized them because they all looked emaciated. They each took out a packed lunch of greens — *just* greens — and a small kitchen scale and proceeded to weigh the lettuce before sprinkling it with a bit of vinegar. None of them looked healthy and vibrant, and the younger ones looked like they might be prematurely aging. One young man in particular adamantly defended caloric restriction, and I gently tried to broaden his perspective.

"You know, one of the things you're doing is exchanging reproduction for longevity," I said.

"No, that's not true," he said. "We can have reproduction."

The others nodded.

"Do you know your testosterone level?" I asked him.

"Two hundred."

"Well, that's very low. How do you think you'll have reproduction?"

"Because I can stop this at any time."

"No, because when you have low testosterone, you don't have desire. You're not going to have the *desire* to stop. I have longevity because my genes are in my kids already. My DNA may live forever, but you're only going to have your life span. Maybe you think it'll be long, but not if you're killing yourself."

I don't run into CRONies as often as I used to, so maybe they are adopting healthier approaches to eating.

AGING BEGINS
BEFORE WE'RE BORN

One of the biggest surprises we've had regarding aging in the past few decades is that aging begins in utero. This hypothesis by David Barker, a British epidemiologist, proposed that slow intrauterine growth, low birth weight, and premature birth have a relationship with the origins of diseases that typically show up in middle age, including hypertension, coronary heart disease, and type 2 diabetes.

Barker's theory is based on observations he made of people who had been born in an area of the Netherlands near the end of World War II, when the food supply was extremely low. The women who were pregnant at that time gave birth to small babies, and when those children were very young, they already had a high incidence of age-related diseases, including diabetes, hypertension, and kidney failure. Barker's hypothesis was that they had protected themselves while in utero to survive with minimal calories but that when they were born and had enough to eat, that survival strategy had an adverse effect. Somehow, getting a normal amount of nutrition was actually harming them.

In a study at Einstein, a team of obstetricians, Francine Einstein and Hye Jung Heo, and geneticist John Greally Reid Thompson and I showed that young rats that were small for their age had an epigenetic methylation profile that was similar to those of old rats, linking the mechanism of aging as a result of small birth and epigenetic mechanisms. In separate human studies, they also showed that babies who are born small have different epigenetic methylation patterns than average-size babies. These studies and others indicate that some aging depends on the conditions that exist in utero and continues throughout stages of life. So scratches on the CD start the aging process before we're even born.

SuperAgers' Top Secrets

So far, we've discovered three primary traits that SuperAgers have in common. Not all SuperAgers have all three, but these three phenomena most profoundly slow aging — and offer hope for the rest of us.

1. **High levels of good cholesterol**
   HDL — high-density lipoprotein — cholesterol protects from heart attacks and dementia.
2. **Unusually low levels of the growth hormone IGF-1**

This protein produced in the liver helps to grow tissue. Low IGF-1 helps us shift our energy from growth to survival.

3. **Unusually high levels of some MDPs**

These proteins originate in the mitochondria and have many varieties — some of which are found *only* in SuperAgers — that build resilience against the stresses of aging.

Along with giving us some great leads to follow, our research with SuperAgers has made it clear that we need to follow exceptional longevity over years and decades. Though we have learned a lot with our Longevity Genes Project and made important observations and connections, studying people at a certain age provides only a fragment of the information we can get by following them throughout life. With that in mind, we launched a new study called Lon-Genity, for which we recruited Ashkenazi Jews whose parents had lived to be ninety-five or older and who were not already in our LGP project. This group is called OPEL — offspring of parents with exceptional longevity — while our control group is called OPUS — offspring of parents with usual survival. We have nearly fourteen hundred people in the study, and we are doing a vast amount of testing on them every year, including extensive neurocognitive tests, MRIs of their brains, and CT scans of their coronary arteries. We're trying to capture detailed information about their health as they grow old and, of course, find the relationship between their health and the longevity genes. The long-term objectives are to identify genes that contribute to exceptional longevity in humans and assess associations among these genes, age-related diseases, and longevity.

To date, our research results have been encouraging and enthusiastically received by the medical research community. Among the findings, the team has learned that longevity is:

- highly likely to be inherited from generation to generation;
- highly correlated to high levels of HDL cholesterol and low levels of LDL — low-density lipoprotein ("bad") — cholesterol; and
- likely to occur among people with larger HDL and LDL molecule sizes, which results in lower incidence of

cardiovascular disease, insulin resistance, and hypertension.

Three:
Cholesterol:
Is More Better?

In the decades that I have been studying the cholesterol levels of centenarians' plasma, I have also been studying aging in animals that get different types of diseases than people but age similarly. All animals age in similar manners — skin, hair, skeletal bones, and muscle all change shape and function, and diseases are contracted more frequently. Finding out what is and is not fundamental to aging in a wide variety of organisms was crucial for cracking the code of human longevity. Studying different organisms has helped us to put together a true picture of what aging necessarily *is* for humans — and what elements are inessential and can be avoided. For example, my friend Steven N. Austad, author of *Why We Age,* studied clams that were five hundred years old and small invertebrate organisms called *hydra* that don't seem to age at all. And Vera Gorbunova and her husband,

Andrei Seluanov, investigate why the naked mole rat lives up to twenty times longer than any other rodent.

By comparing the results of our animal studies with the information we collected from centenarians, we are progressively cracking the code of how to slow aging for us all. Yet humans are special, and our cholesterol metabolism is different from that of many animals, particularly rodents. As it turned out, our first clue about the link between cholesterol and longevity came from centenarians. Cholesterol is a type of fat that is in our blood and builds every cell of our bodies. Without it, we would not develop and would probably die, but many people still think of it as a harmful substance that we only get from eating certain foods like meat, eggs, fish, and dairy products. These foods do contain cholesterol, but you might be surprised to hear that it's your body weight that has the biggest effect on your blood levels of cholesterol. You also may not know that the liver is central in co-ordinating the metabolism of cholesterol and moving it through the body. Cholesterol is also leaving our bodies through the secretion of bile that begins in the liver. This co-ordination is important for thousands of biological functions, mainly for cells' membrane layer and production of hormones such as vitamin D. But despite being a vital organic molecule, cholesterol has managed to earn a questionable reputation.

The lipid panel that is part of a standard annual checkup shows the levels of HDL and LDL cholesterols, which make up most of our cholesterol. The lipid panel also shows the level of triglycerides (TG), which makes up about 20 percent of total cholesterol. In clinical practice, your doctor may be more concerned with the ratio between the LDL and the HDL than with the individual numbers. If the ratio is smaller than 3:1, your doctor may not be worried about your LDL number even if it's higher.

Before these numbers were commonly broken out in test results, the total cholesterol number was misleading, and fat became our archenemy because it was linked to high cholesterol, which increases our risk for cardiovascular disease. But we need fat for our brains and other organs to function, so the total cholesterol number is not nearly as relevant as the individual levels of each type of cholesterol. For example, when we have high LDL, we have a greater risk of heart disease because it combines with fat, calcium, and other substances to form plaque in our arteries. This buildup, called *atherosclerosis,* constricts the flow of oxygen-rich blood to the heart and other organs. When we decrease LDL, we get less heart disease and significantly lower our chances of dying from symptoms of the disease, including heart attacks. On the other hand, having high levels of HDL seems to protect us from heart disease. And women tend to have higher levels of HDL than men, so that may also be a factor in why they live longer than men on average. Although when people ask me why husbands often die before their wives, I say, "Because they want to." I'm kidding, of course, and statistics show that married men live longer, on average, than men who are not married.

We often see high levels of triglycerides in people who are obese, and being obese increases the risk of type 2 diabetes, heart disease, and strokes. Type 2 diabetes patients have varying levels of LDL, but they usually have high triglycerides and low HDL. Not surprisingly, most of the cholesterol studies conducted to date have explored the connection between cholesterol and cardiovascular disease, and the conclusions have led to the development of the class of drugs called *statins* that were designed to prevent heart attacks. Statins, such as Lipitor and

Crestor, lower bad cholesterol by moderating how much of it the liver produces, how much circulates in the bloodstream, and how much is secreted through the bile duct and into our intestines.

When statins were tested in clinical trials, they prevented heart attacks and death from heart attacks by 25–30 percent, compared with people not taking them. On the other hand, statins usually did not change overall mortality even though heart diseases play such a large role in mortality. How can these drugs prevent the major contributor to death but not result in less death overall? I was an author of one of the first three studies showing that people who are on statins have a 30 percent higher risk of developing type 2 diabetes than people who aren't, and some research has suggested that using statins also increases the likelihood of suicide. I was also concerned that lowering LDL cholesterol too much would be harmful to the neurons in the brain, some of the richest cholesterol-containing cells in our bodies. While extremely low LDL has recently been associated with bleeding strokes, the literature generally does not suggest negative effects, maybe because its anti-atherosclerosis effects are in balance with the need for cholesterol for better brain function in the elderly. Whatever the case, while there can be drawbacks to taking statins, overall they are making a big difference for millions of people who have not been able to lower their LDL cholesterol levels without them.

So from the standpoint of being a specific drug treatment that targets a specific human disease, statin therapy is helpful, but on average, it does not increase longevity in humans or animals, and it may be unnecessary and even unsafe in people eighty or older who have cardiovascular disease. Statin therapy is very different from aging therapy, which is what we are most interested in at Einstein. That's why when we looked at cholesterol in SuperAgers and their offspring, we looked at it through a different lens.

UNLOCKING CHOLESTEROL'S LONGEVITY SECRETS

When we began finding centenarians for our Longevity Genes Project, we conducted basic tests similar to those you would undergo at an annual checkup, which include measuring electrolyte and glucose levels, checking kidney functions, and drawing blood to do a lipid panel. In a diverse population, men's HDL cholesterol levels average about 45 mg/dl and women's average about 55, but the centenarians' offspring sometimes had HDL levels over 100! The centenarians themselves had HDL levels in the 50s, which isn't considered high, but when you take into account that HDL decreases by about five points every eight years starting at middle age, their HDL would have been expected to be around 20. For example, Eva Fleischer's mother, Muti, was 102 and had HDL cholesterol of 62, which is at the upper end of the average range for a woman at that age, and Eva herself had HDL cholesterol of 142 mg/dl. Now that our study has grown, we have many people with HDL that's above 100, which is a remarkable phenotype because very few people have HDL that's 80 or above. If a man's HDL is 60 and a woman's HDL is 70, it's considered fabulous.

An interesting side story involving this data is that when HDL is measured in the general population, the average across all ages is always about 45 for men and about 55 for women. But how is this possible if, individually, it goes down five points every eight years when we follow up with the same subjects? My explanation is that when the HDL goes down, it stops protecting against the consequences of aging, and people die.

The average is maintained in the population because HDL is a survival factor. While centenarians have average HDL levels, we know from their offspring that their HDL was probably much higher when they were seventy or eighty. And we are worried that those with lower HDL may be at risk for dying in the coming year or so.

The connection between high HDL and exceptional longevity was clear, but we didn't know what caused it. To find out, we began by looking more closely at the centenarians' blood. How might it be different from those in the control group? What we found astonished us. These fatty cholesterol molecules are often packaged into larger clusters and transported through the body in the blood. In the case of the centenarians and their offspring, they didn't only have more HDL but had much larger HDL and LDL particles than average. Larger HDL and LDL particles are associated with decreased risk of hypertension, cardiovascular disease, and metabolic syndrome. In fact, it is believed that small particles easily oxidize and are a ready template for initiating the first steps of atherosclerosis. And as it turned out, some people in the control group who did not have hypertension or cardiovascular disease also had HDL and

LDL particles that were significantly larger than average.

Part of the reason for the higher HDL levels in our centenarians is that they are packed on specific carriers — APOA — that transport more cholesterol than normal away from the arteries. While centenarians' LDL levels are usually normal, their LDL tends to be in formations that are larger than average, and they have their own specific carriers — APOB — to move the "loads." These larger forms undergo less oxidation than smaller ones, so they are less likely to form the plaque that causes atherosclerosis. So it's confusing, because it is hard to tell whether the cholesterol profile of centenarians is because of their total HDL, the ratio of LDL to HDL, the large HDL particle sizes, the large LDL particle sizes, or a combination of some or all of the above. Whatever the reason, centenarians with one or more of these characteristics have less heart disease, less chance of Alzheimer's, greater cognitive function, and — of course — longer lives. Whatever the case, the bigger question was: What was responsible for these differences?

We continued to search for the answer, but the high levels of good cholesterol were so consistent that now when I see patients with high HDL and longevity in the family, my thought is that they are "at risk" of living a long time. While most of my time is devoted to research and educating people about our findings, I have volunteered at the Bronx's Montefiore Diabetes Clinic for the past twenty-seven years, and one patient of mine stands out regarding cholesterol levels. She was a fifty-eight-year-old woman who, despite her diabetes, seemed to be in remarkably good health. One strange piece of the puzzle was that she had an HDL cholesterol level far above normal. For a woman of her age, especially with her illness, we would expect her HDL cholesterol levels to be 35 to 45. Instead, she clocked in at 100! She looked at least a decade younger than her age, while her husband was a decade younger than she was but looked much older. In my experience, the difference between chronological and biological aging was never more striking than in this couple, who looked like they were twenty years apart but the younger-looking one was actually older.

"I know this sounds strange," I said when I met her, "but I have to ask — do you have any unusually old people in your family?"

Her eyes widened. "Well, yes!" she said. "My mother is 96 years old and doing well.

And her father lived to 114. How did you know?"

I told her about our longevity study and said that centenarians and their families have unusually high levels of HDL cholesterol, especially when compared with their average LDL cholesterol levels. By this point, I was quite comfortable treating this phenomenon as a real indicator of longevity.

ARE THERE REALLY GOOD GENE MUTATIONS?

After seeing similar cholesterol results in hundreds of centenarians and offspring, we were convinced that whatever was responsible for their differences could be inherited. So we began looking for cholesterol genes that might have significant mutations that were doing good instead of harm. But we ran into some unanticipated resistance from the IRB because the members were concerned about what we would do if we discovered people who had harmful mutations that caused diseases. If we happen to see one, there isn't anything we can do about it.

Discovering mutations and variants is exciting, but the findings are given the same weight as the findings of association studies until we can validate them in other populations or do functional studies on cells or animals to prove that the mutations are important.

Once we got approval from the IRB for our study, we began looking at a variety of genes that are associated with the creation and transportation of cholesterol, and we discovered that two genes that modulate HDL cholesterol and triglycerides had functional variants, meaning that the genes functioned differently because of the mutation. And many of our centenarians had one or two genetic variants that affect the clustering of the cholesterol particles:

- About 18 percent of our centenarians have a specific variant in a gene called *cholesteryl ester transfer protein* (CETP) that's associated with high HDL and with longevity. This variation inhibits the action of CETP.
- About 20 percent of our centenarians have a mutation in the APOC3 gene, one of the carriers of HDL cholesterol, in the gene's "promoter" region — the "switch" that turns the gene on and off — which results in higher good cholesterol and lower triglycerides.

Both of these variations are giving us insights into cardiovascular health and longevity, and we're delighted that our findings have helped two pharmaceutical companies develop inhibitor-type drugs. One of the reasons for failures in drug development is that we assume we know what to expect in humans based on what we learn from mice. For pharmaceutical development, it is important to first find people who have mutations or variants in the gene that the company wants to target. They want to see variants or mutations that either cause a disease or prevent it. Furthermore, if the mutation or the variant causes the exact effect that the company wants to mimic, they will want to see if there are downsides to the variant, so there's a need to gather data on safety. In our case, both variants were more common in centenarians than in the unrelated control group, and that was a good sign that they were safe. The pharmaceutical companies were not really interested in the variants' potential for the treatment of aging but in their potential for the prevention of coronary heart diseases. In the near future, though, we *will* have pharmaceuticals that mimic these variants so that everyone can enjoy the health benefits and the extra years.

SOLVING THE MYSTERY OF
HELPFUL GENE MUTATIONS

The cholesteryl ester transfer protein gene plays an essential role in regulating cholesterol. However, the function of the variants causing a decrease in CETP action is not fully understood. On one hand, like a shuttle bus, it transfers the cholesteryl ester from the coronary vessels of the heart and out of the body through the bile and intestines. The mutation inhibits the carrier from disposing of the cholesterol, so why would you want to develop a drug that stops the shuttle of bad cholesterol? On the other hand, because the load of cholesterol is not getting off its transporter, the particles become bigger and bigger, and this may be the pivotal effect. Maybe the fact that the particles become larger and packed together prevents damage to the vessels. So while a decrease in CETP can have both benefits and drawbacks, the good appears to outweigh the bad.

There are indications that the mutation in CETP may protect us from heart disease, which is wonderful, but at Einstein, we wanted to know if it goes so far as to protect us from aging and therefore from more than one disease. If we could determine that it does, we could say that CETP is a longevity gene, not a disease gene. So we looked at this mutation to see what other age-related diseases it might affect, and we found that it is associated with protection from hypertension. Granted, one could argue that hypertension is part of cardiovascular disease, but it is also an age-related condition.

We also looked at all the subjects in our study who had the variants to see if they had less prevalence of cancer than those without the variants. As it turned out, they did not, maybe because we don't have that many cancers in our SuperAgers population, but we saw that the people with this mutation developed cancer an average of ten years later than people without the CETP mutation. Though that was just an observation — without enough subjects and statistical power to call it significant — it gave us the sense that the variants we were finding that led to high HDL would also provide other protections from other age-related diseases and therefore are targeting a basic biology of aging.

But the biggest prize for us will always be cognitive preservation. Is there a link between the mutation and cognitive decline? Our own data showed that centenarians with the CETP mutation had experienced a small fraction of the cognitive decline of centenarians who did not have the mutation. Moreover, we had a couple of subjects who had a major gene risk for Alzheimer's called *APOE4.* The textbooks suggest that carriers of the gene will have dementia at age seventy and be dead at eighty, but our subjects did not have dementia and were still alive at *one hundred.* Both of these subjects had the CETP mutation.

To validate our findings regarding the link between the mutation and cognitive decline, we collaborated with Richard Lipton, a professor of neurology, epidemiology, and population health who is leading the Einstein Aging Study. This study recruited hundreds of people between the ages of forty-five and sixty-five and followed their cognition over three decades. The researchers looked for changes in cognition and attempted to formulate physical or biological tests that could predict decline. They genotyped the CETP variant of the CETP gene in the participants and demonstrated that those who had it experienced 70 percent less incidence of Alzheimer's and cognitive decline. The study subjects were mostly white, but there were also some Jews and some blacks, and the protective factors for black people were the most striking. There is no other example of a single variant that extends this magnitude of protection against cognitive decline or Alzheimer's disease.

But our findings have not been confirmed by all the studies that have been done. For example, in a study of centenarians conducted in southern Italy, there wasn't a greater presence of the CETP variants in the centenarians than in the rest of the population, so we did not get validation from that study. In northern Italy, however, the same study was done with a group of Italian centenarians who were genetically different from those in the south, and the results were similar to ours, showing that there was greater longevity and protection against Alzheimer's disease among those with the variants. But then David Bennett, the star of Alzheimer's disease research at Rush University, tested our variant in his study and showed that, if anything, the people with the CETP mutation in his study had cognitive function that was not as good as the cognitive function in the control group. The difference was relatively small, but we *are* seeing that we get different results in different populations.

What we've learned is that when you have a single variant and you look at it in isolation, you can't always validate it, because populations are not made of a single variant; they are made from many variants, and some cancel each other out. For example, in our study, the centenarians and their offspring who had the CETP variant and high HDL levels are likely to have longevity, but if you have a population that has the mutation but doesn't have high HDL, they probably will not have longevity. So it is not enough to look at the variant — we have to look at the phenotype of the variants, which in this case is HDL.

Not long after we made the discovery about the CETP variant, Pfizer began developing a CETP inhibitor that was intended to work the same way the variant worked in our centenarians. The study was shut down soon after it began, because people who had taken the drug experienced a substantial increase in blood pressure and therefore more cardiovascular events instead of fewer. It turned out that the drug had more than one action, so it was not only inhibiting the CETP but also affecting other systems. Once it was understood that this was not a mechanistic error but a bad drug development, Merck & Co. considered continuing the development of its own CETP inhibitor, and the company was receptive to seeing our results. I imagine that it received input from more studies than ours, but our study is the only one that showed that people with this mutation live to be one hundred, which at least means that targeting CETP is very safe.

I suggested that Merck also do a cognitive function assessment of people with the CETP variation. The assessment did not indicate that the people in the study were protected against cognitive decline, but that may have been because they were a much younger population than we tested in our study, and they used a test that is much less sensitive for people that age. So we're not sure if the CETP variant preserves cognitive function or not. Because our centenarians had these mutations before they were born, maybe the effects we're seeing began when they were children or in their twenties or forties and fifties. If that's the case, then giving the drug to people in their sixties or older may not work. To find the answer to when the drug might optimally be taken, we need to study cognition longitudinally, because even with very sophisticated tests, we usually don't see cognitive decline in people until they are seventy or older even when they have been diagnosed with Alzheimer's.

But what's even more significant than the individual studies is that when we have a group of people with variants or mutations that protect from or cause certain diseases, pharmaceutical companies can use this knowledge to develop drugs that target those genes to either inhibit their functions or activate them to prevent or treat diseases. The best example of this so far is a gene called *PCSK9*. Human research studies showed in 2003 that a gain-of-function mutation — a mutation that results in new or stronger protein function — causes familial hyperlipidemia, abnormally high levels of fats in the blood. Amazingly enough, by 2006, there was a study that showed that a loss-of-function mutation — a mutation that results in less or no protein function — brought an 88 percent reduction in coronary heart diseases. Then, in 2012, *The New England Journal of Medicine* published a study looking at a population who had the protective variant for PCSK9. It found that the effects of inhibiting the enzyme over a longer time reduced the risk of cardiovascular disease without creating the adverse effect of blocking this pathway. Then in 2018, *The New England Journal of Medicine* published the phase-three study on the PCSK9 inhibitor evolocumab (Repatha) and alirocumab (Praluent). In one of the studies, among patients who had a previous acute coronary syndrome and were treated with statins, the risk of recurrent ischemic cardiovascular events — in which blood flow to the heart is obstructed — was lower among those who received evolocumab than among those who received a placebo.

With this valuable genetic information, researchers didn't need to spend years doing animal research, so it took relatively little time for alirocumab to be developed as the new therapy for people who cannot tolerate statins or need additional help.

THE BENEFITS OF CETP
PERSONIFIED

Irving Kahn didn't work until the end of his life. He just worked until he was 108. In late 2014, just a year before he died at 109, he finally retired as chairman of the Wall Street investment firm Kahn Brothers, which he founded in 1978 with two of his sons and which manages between $800 million and $900 million in assets. Until then, he reviewed every proposed transaction and had the final word on investment policy from the firm's corner office. The idea of not working was unthinkable to Irving.

"If you took it away from me, I'd try to buy it back," he said during one of my visits with him. Age 104 at the time, he also told me that his exceptional longevity had its advantages in the business world. "You know what's rotten and what's fresh and what's good or bad, and you can participate at a higher level of successful choices. That's me."

"Work is his life," his son Thomas, company president, said at the time. "He's always been an absorber of information. Ever since I was a child, he would bring home annual reports and read them at the dinner table, and that's what he still does." The family believes that work also probably did more than anything else to help Irving through his grief after the death of his wife, Ruth, in 1996 after sixty-five years of marriage.

Thomas thinks his father's passion for work came from an appetite for knowledge. Irving read three newspapers a day and constantly added to his personal library of thousands of books, most of them about scientific developments and possibilities.

"The important thing is to keep the brain going, you see," he said.

Speaking of the brain, Irving was a progressive thinker when it came to social issues and philanthropy. One of his favorite causes was the Jewish Foundation for Education of Women, for which he was a trustee emeritus. He also founded the New York City Job and Career Center in 1986 to help prepare high school students for the workforce.

Hand in hand with his social consciousness was a sense of his own empowerment, which he ultimately credits to his parents. Irving's mother had her own shirtwaist business, and his father taught him to ride a bike by giving him a single push. "He said, 'Stay on this street and hold on to the handlebars,' and gave me a push. Well, here I was out in the middle of the street . . . What could I do? So I learned how to ride pretty quickly." His father used a similar approach to teach Irving how to swim. "He pushed me in the water and said, 'Would you rather die or rather swim?' "

It wouldn't be much of an exaggeration to say Irving had been his own man ever since. He began his Wall Street career in 1928, and despite having only a year's experience by the time of the stock crash in 1929, he managed to turn a profit while so many others lost everything.

As speculation ran rampant that summer, Irving realized that short selling was the road to success. Under that strategy, he would profit from a fall in the price of a stock rather than a rise. His first stock trade was a short sale in a copper mining company, and an in-law lent him the money for it despite his certainty that Irving would lose his shirt by betting against the bull market.

Well, Irving proved him wrong by almost doubling his money when the crash hit.

Before long, though, he adopted the much more conservative approach known as *value investing,* which he learned from the creator of the concept, Benjamin Graham, at Columbia University in the 1930s. (Warren Buffett was also a disciple of Graham's, and Irving and Buffett would ride the subway to his lectures together, Thomas says.) Under the value investing strategy, investors assess a stock's actual value and buy shares only if they are available for a significantly lower price. It's the strategy that saw Kahn Brothers through the crash of 2008 and multiple sell-offs over the past forty-plus years. And it saw *Irving* through more than eight decades of crashes, beginning with the big one.

In a 2014 interview with *The Daily Telegraph* of London, Irving summed up the philosophy that has been Kahn Brothers' guiding light:

There are always good companies that are overpriced. A disciplined investor avoids them. As Warren Buffett has correctly said, a good investor has the opposite temperament to that prevailing in the market. Throughout all the crashes, sticking to value investing helped me to preserve and grow my capital. Investors must remember that their first job is to preserve their capital. After they've dealt with that, they can approach the second job, seeking a return on the capital . . . Our goal has always been to seek reasonable returns over a very long period of time. I don't know why anyone would look at a short time horizon. In my life, I invested over decades . . . I prefer to be slow and steady.

The value investing strategy that Irving helped to pioneer seems to reflect his practical approach to life in general. He led a modest lifestyle and didn't see the sense in spending more on life's necessities than was necessary. His wardrobe was a good example. To the office, he would wear a purely functional oxford shirt with a conservative tie, and he'd put on a bright blue fleece vest if he felt a chill. He also went to bed at eight and got up at seven like clockwork, and he was diligent about taking his vitamins.

When asked if he thought his sensible approach to life had something to do with his longevity, he'd say, "Maybe." When asked if he thought it was likelier genetic, he'd say no and politely explain that he wasn't interested in the reason for his longevity. Fortunately, though, he was willing to participate in Einstein's Longevity Genes Project.

Thomas backs the argument for genetics, saying Irving's diet was far from healthy, including many more cheeseburgers than salads. And then there was Irving's older sister, Helen Reichert, who lived to be 110 and smoked for more than *ninety* of those years. (So again, we see centenarians being protected from habits that are very unhealthy for most people.)

When Irving died, the obituary headlines called him the world's oldest stockbroker, and the stories all mentioned that he was one of the few people who have celebrated their one-hundredth birthdays by ringing the opening bell at the New York Stock Exchange.

A Mutation That Adds Years to Life Span?

In addition to the CETP mutation, in 2006, we discovered that some of our centenarians had a mutation in the APOC3 gene, which is found on triglyceride-rich lipoprotein, and that these centenarians had lower triglycerides and higher HDL cholesterol. The association of this mutation with longevity is so powerful that even among centenarians, it appears to add a year to their lives on average. Triglycerides increase our risk for cardiovascular diseases and are typically high in people who are obese or have type 2 diabetes. These types of study results are why controlling cholesterol is becoming one of the top ways to target aging (even if we can't formally call it that just yet) while increasing overall health.

My colleague Alan Shuldiner made similar discoveries with the link between APOC3 and longevity in an Amish population in 2008. He found that the Amish have a mutation in the same gene but in a different location. The people in his study who had this loss-of-function mutation had fewer heart attacks and lived longer than average, but none of them made it to one hundred. In 2014, two additional populations with the same mutation demonstrated about a

40 percent reduction in coronary heart diseases. So there has been a lot of validation of the protective nature of mutations in APOC3, and fortunately, the company Ionis developed a drug that inhibits APOC3 and changes the lipid panel to lower triglycerides and raise HDL. It completed a phase-three trial in 2015, so this drug will soon be available. Just to be clear, as with Merck's development of a CETP inhibitor, Ionis is not developing this drug to target aging — they're interested in targeting diseases. But the fact that centenarians have this mutation is a good indication that it's safe.

Our research and treatments are the greatest possible argument for preventive medicine. Just like managing the flu or rickets, targeting aging is good for society, our economy, and our politics. As former U.S. senator Claire McCaskill noted when we met with her about the dividends of having people stay healthy longer, even reducing adult diabetes by a "modest" percentage could evaporate our national debt. The longer and healthier we all live, the better, safer, and more prosperous we can be as a society.

The Italians like to toast, *"Cent'anni,"* which has come to mean "May you live for a hundred years." The comparable Jewish blessing is "May you live until 120," which is the number of years that Moses lived. Once, such sentiments were just wishful thinking, but perhaps now they will become the new normal. For now, though, we can stick to the humbler but wonderfully joyful Hebrew toast: *l'chaim* — to life.

FOUR:
GROWTH HORMONES:
LESS IS MORE

If you want to look and feel younger, Be Younger Tomorrow is what you've been waiting for. Why settle for the fat, the wrinkles, the loss of muscle strength and the declining libido that come with age when you can turn everything around with just one capsule a day? This revolutionary treatment contains human growth hormone, so what are you waiting for? The fountain of youth is just a phone call away. But call now. Supplies are limited.

(These statements have not been evaluated by the Food and Drug Administration.)

These kinds of claims have not been evaluated, let alone approved by the FDA, because there's no credible scientific proof to support them. Rather, the research shows that increasing the levels of growth hormones can do quite a bit of harm. The natural decline of growth hormones that occurs with aging is not considered a deficiency, and in cases where there *is* an actual growth hormone deficiency, the patients are treated with injections, not pills, because the hormone simply disintegrates when it's eaten; it is not absorbed through the intestines as it would need to be in order to be effective.

In Lucas Cranach the Elder's 1546 painting *Fountain of Youth,* old women enter a pool of water and emerge as younger women. That's a tall order, and if we're ever to reverse aging, we first need to figure out how to *stop* it, let alone slow it, which is exactly what geroscientists are trying to do. While the idea of boosting levels of growth hormones to slow aging was interesting, we have learned that although growth hormones are essential *as* we're growing, in general they may cause harm from the perspective of aging. If growth hormones decline with age, we first need to consider if rushing to reverse this is benefiting or protecting us. As I mentioned in chapter 2, the natural decline of some hormones works as a protective mechanism, so boosting hormone levels is a serious affair.

LESS GROWTH MAY LEAD TO AN EXCEPTIONALLY LONG LIFE

On the surface, the connection between fewer growth hormones and longevity seems contradictory, because when we look at the relationship between body size and longevity, the bigger the animal species, the longer its life span. But we see something totally different when we look *within* each species. Small dogs live longer than big dogs, ponies live longer than horses, and mice born with a genetic defect that causes dwarfism live substantially longer than mice without this defect. We wondered if this holds true for human beings, too, specifically our centenarians.

Although growth is important for the species, it's an energetic process that requires extensive resources, so stopping growth early extends health span and life span in nearly every species that has been studied. When we modulate the growth hormone genes in animals, those with lower levels of growth hormones live longer than those with higher levels. For example, Andrzej Bartke, professor of internal medicine at Southern Illinois University, conducted endocrinology research in which he studied mice that were dwarf models and whose major problem was growth hormone deficiency. He connected this deficiency to longevity, and while I found his model interesting, I wasn't convinced, because the effects of a growth hormone called *insulin-like growth factor 1* (IGF-1) on humans can be both beneficial and detrimental. On one hand, high levels of IGF-1 are associated with an increase in many types of cancers. But on the other hand, high IGF-1 levels have been associated with improved cognition, glucose tolerance, and muscle and cardiovascular function.

Growth hormone is secreted by the pituitary gland, which is located at the base of the brain, right behind the nose. It binds to cell receptors and stimulates growth as well as the reproduction and regeneration of cells. When growth hormones bind to receptors in the liver, the liver secretes another important growth and maintenance hormone called *insulin-like growth factor* 1 (IGF-1). IGF-1 has receptors throughout the body through which many of the functions of growth hormones are achieved.

At Einstein, we had been studying IGF-1 in another context. We were looking at the brains of rats, specifically the hypothalamus, which regulates the secretion of hormones from the pituitary but is also a master regulator of other functions, such as appetite, metabolism, and reproduction. Regarding metabolism, when we eat, glucose causes the secretion of insulin from specific cells in the pancreas to keep levels of glucose within the normal range. Insulin also inhibits the "meltdown" of fat that is used for energy when we're fasting, and it suppresses production of glucose from the liver. What we discovered is that all the effects that occur after we eat can be modulated by directly manipulating the hypothalamus with insulin and other hormones. So we wondered if IGF-1 could also control glucose metabolism in the rest of the body, directly through the hypothalamus.

To find out, Radhika Muzumdar, a pediatric endocrinologist at Einstein, infused small doses of human IGF-1 to rats' brains, right next to the hypothalamus. The IGF-1 suppressed the production of glucose from the liver through its action on the hypothalamus. So the answer was yes — higher levels of IGF-1 in the brain mimicked insulin's effect in the rest of body, and it did so without

153

IGF-1's "spilling" into the bloodstream. Derek Huffman, associate professor of molecular pharmacology and medicine and the director of Health Span Core at Einstein's Nathan Shock Center, achieved the same results with aging rats that were achieved with young rats. But dwarf rodents with low IGF-1 live longer than those that are not dwarfs, without having metabolic problems, so we wondered how IGF-1 could be good and bad at the same time.

We decided to take a close look at the effects of a pathway that includes hundreds of biological proteins that are involved in the regulation of growth called the *GH/IGF-1 axis.* The hypothesis was that functional genetic variants in growth hormones and the IGF-1 axis contribute to the longevity of centenarians.

GROWTH HORMONE CLUES
FROM OUR CENTENARIANS

Once we had a reasonable number of centenarians in our study, I recruited the best functional geneticist in the field of human aging, Yousin Suh. Yousin was interested in studying GH/IGF-1's pathways, and she came up with a system to gather as much significant information from the centenarians as possible for the lowest cost possible.

She began by studying the top dozen genes on our list of the hundreds of genes that are involved in the growth hormone/IGF-1 pathways. She studied the DNA of many of those genes and found that some sequences had many changes and others, such as the IGF-1 gene itself, had practically no changes. She went from gene to gene, and we finally got a direct hit; the significant difference was not with IGF-1 itself but in its receptor, IGF-1R.

Genetic defects can occur in genes' receptors as well as the genes themselves, and so far, we have not found significant mutations in the IGF-1 gene. But in nine of the centenarians (2 percent of the number we had gathered by that time), we found two kinds of mutations that had never been discovered on the receptor for IGF-1. What's more, these centenarians were shorter by an inch than centenarians without the mutations. (People sometimes ask what the average height was, but that's not relevant to most people, because our study group tends to be shorter than the general population, the average height is different for men and women, and people lose height as they age, so we were comparing maximal heights.)

At about the same time, Martin Holzenberger, a French biologist, found that when he deleted *all* the IGF-1 receptors from the chromosomes that carry the gene from the eggs of the pregnant mice, the pups were stillborn. That's how important the effects of IGF-1 are, and its absence cannot be compensated for by other mechanisms. However, when he deleted only half of the IGF-1 receptors, the mice were born. Although those mice were 20 percent smaller than the others, they lived significantly longer than mice that had all the IGF-1 receptors, with the effect on longevity being much greater in females. So we learned that examples of mutations in IGF-1 receptors and longevity exist throughout nature.

To determine whether the centenarians' cells with the mutations in the IGF-1 receptors would have the impaired function that we suspected they would, my dear friend Pinchas "Hassy" Cohen, dean of USC Leonard Davis School of Gerontology, studied cells with and without the mutations. He demonstrated that our suspicions were correct — the cells with the mutations block the effects of IGF-1. But nobody in the original control group had the mutations, and when we wanted to publish a paper on this study, the statistical reviewer

THE FOREVER CELLS

At Einstein, we routinely "immortalize" our centenarians' cells so that we have unlimited DNA to draw on in our experiments. The process involves turning lymphocytes — the type of white blood cells that are recruited to fight viral infections — into cancer cells known as *lymphoblasts,* which are immortal, and freezing them. We can defrost parts of cells and grow more DNA. So the cells of the centenarians in our study are alive and will be contributing to scientific discoveries long after they leave us.

noted that a statistical comparison when compared with zero does not exist. So we expanded the control group and tested many more people until Yousin found someone with one of the receptor mutations. Finally, our results were statistically legitimate, and we could publish the paper, adding to the evidence that functional modulation of the GH/IGF-1 pathway affects longevity across nature — including humans. We had our first proof that a cluster of people may have increased health span and life span because of an impaired function in the action of a gene that was caused by a single variation, just as we had seen in animal studies.

Although other mutations in the GH/IGF-1 axis have been found in people with exceptional longevity around the world, the mutations in the IGF-1 receptors we found have been seen only in AJs. But I still wasn't convinced that finding it in 2 percent of our centenarians was compelling enough. Maybe those people were specifically protected only from cancer, which improved their chances of living long lives, and were not protected from other diseases.

Meanwhile, our geneticist Gil Atzmon looked at a severe deletion in the sequence of the growth hormone receptor (GHR) that had been discovered in a low percentage of people around the world. The action of growth hormone on its receptors has several functions, but of course, we were interested in how much IGF-1 the liver would secrete into our subjects' bloodstreams. Gil found that 12 percent of our male centenarians had this deletion of an entire exon (an area of a gene that codes for protein) known as *d3GHR,* while only 3–4 percent of our control group had it. The overrepresentation in the centenarians suggested that it could be a longevity genotype, so we had yet another lead to follow. If this deletion did affect growth hormone function and in particular the production of IGF-1, then growth hormone would not be able to produce sufficient IGF-1 from the liver.

And indeed, when we measured IGF-1 levels in our affected centenarians, they had significantly lower levels of IGF-1 than those without the deletion. So it stood to reason that since they had had this mutation throughout their lives, they should also be shorter than the centenarians without the mutation. But that's where we ran into a mystery that delayed publication of our study results for nearly a decade — the affected centenarians were significantly *taller* than those without the mutation! But why?

Gil decided to see if he could validate his studies in populations other than AJs to find out if the deletion exists among them and, if so, if there is greater incidence among the oldest subjects. He reached out to three groups that were conducting aging studies, and in all three of them, the people with exceptional longevity had an overrepresentation in this deletion. This validation was exciting, and I was convinced that it was a significant discovery, but there was still the problem of explaining how this alteration resulted in our affected centenarians' being significantly taller than those without the mutation. How could they be taller when the mutation was associated with *less* IGF-1?

When we shared the findings with Hassy, he decided to attempt to solve the mystery by incubating the cells that carried the mutations and measuring the activation of the growth hormone receptor on those cells as well as their ability to proliferate. He found that both activation and ability to proliferate were remarkably stunted. Hassy then repeated the experiment and added excess growth hormone to the cells, and it was as if a switch had been turned on. When stimulated with growth hormones, the same cells that had had less activity showed much higher activation and proliferation than the cells in the control group. Eureka!

The people who were taller than average had grown tall during puberty, when growth hormone levels are very high. Then when growth hormone levels declined after puberty, their receptors were turned down, their cells started producing less IGF-1, and ultimately, their low levels of IGF-1 allowed them to live longer. You can be tall and still have the mutation in the growth hormone axis — and a good shot at exceptional longevity. This also suggests that we may not need to have low IGF-1 action our entire lives; we may be able to get the same benefits by manipulating it later in life.

At the same time as these discoveries regarding the receptor mutations were being made, several groups of people with dwarfism were being studied around the world. Laron dwarfs are a little less than four feet tall, many of them live to be ninety and older, and they all have a mutation that makes the growth hormone receptor inactive. Israeli endocrinologist Zvi Laron — a friend of my father's, whom I met when he chaired the session where I presented my first scientific paper — discovered and studied this syndrome in a group of people in Israel in which closely related Jews become mates. Those who inherit both recessive alleles — or variants of particular genes — from their parents become dwarfs, while siblings who have one normal allele are not born with the disorder. The biggest community of Laron dwarfs is in Ecuador. They are believed to be descendants of Jews who escaped from Spain during the Spanish Inquisition but converted to Christianity to stay alive. Intermarriage within the community explains how recessive genes can get together and cause a syndrome and sometimes a disease.

To study this condition, Dr. Jaime Guevara-Aguirre, the physician who cares for the Laron dwarf population in Ecuador, teamed up with Hassy and Valter Longo, director of USC's Longevity Institute. Their research demonstrated that Laron dwarfs who had the mutation in the growth hormone receptor and, in turn, low levels of IGF-1 had almost no diabetes or cancer — two of the leading age-related diseases. Because of the relatively small number of people affected, the study could not prove that those with the mutation live longer than those who do not, but together with what we have found with our centenarians, the evidence suggests a strong connection between low IGF-1 and longer health span and, in many cases, life span.

We have also been collaborating with groups in other countries that are conducting studies involving people with exceptional longevity. One of the most consistent findings that have resulted from this global collaboration concerns a gene called *FOXO3a*.

Cynthia Kenyon, the biogerontologist (at Calico, LLC) who discovered this gene's equivalent in worms, found that it plays a gatekeeper role in longevity. As it moves in and out of the cell nucleus, it regulates the function of factors like the suppression of tumors and cell death. Meanwhile, geriatrician Bradley Willcox discovered that people with a variant in FOXO3a have better metabolisms and less cardiovascular disease than people without it. In a study that summarized genetic information from many longevity studies, including our own, the frequency in variants of FOXO3a was significantly higher in people with exceptional longevity than in members of control groups.

EPIGENETIC MECHANISMS CAN INCREASE LONGEVITY

Aside from low IGF-1 levels contributing to life span, several epigenetic mechanisms appear to do the same thing, and we expect more of these mechanisms to be discovered. The three main mechanisms we've addressed are:

- **DNA methylation,** a chemical reaction that deactivates some genes and may activate others.
- **Histones,** proteins found in the cell nuclei that package DNA into structural units called *nucleosomes.* They are the primary protein components of

163

chromatin and serve as spools for DNA to wrap around. They also play a role in gene regulation.

- **MicroRNA (or miRNA),** small ribonucleic acid molecules that silence other RNA and thus prevent the expression of certain targeted genes.

Epigenetic mechanisms are responsible in part for how the environment — diet, drugs, environmental chemicals — affects our biology, and they can wreak havoc on our health as we age. For example, if a biochemical methyl group binds to a sequence of DNA as a result of smoking, it can alter the transcription of the DNA, either silencing it (the more common effect) or activating it and potentially putting us at risk for aging and diseases such as cancer. Gil and I acquired a grant to look at methylation's role in longevity — a process that involved studying more than one hundred thousand sites across the DNA where a specific methylation site occurs in many of our centenarians, their offspring, and members of the control group. But when you're trying to make sense of so many changes in methylation sites, you're essentially looking for a needle in a haystack, and sometimes you feel like you're just adding to the haystack.

164

It will take us a while to make sense of all that data because although methylation increases with aging, it occurs in different cells at different times. But a few things are already clear. First, many changes in methylation naturally occur with aging. Second, the methylation patterns of our centenarians' chromosomes are different from the control group's patterns, but some of the methylation sites may get bigger with aging, and some site-specific methylation may protect against aging. Third, the methylation patterns of the centenarians' offspring are somewhere between the centenarians' and the control group's. With the help of these observations, we hope to identify the methylation patterns that are related to longevity. In the meantime, Steve Horvath, a geneticist at UCLA; Morgan Levine, a pathologist at Yale; and a team of others have created what they call a "clock" that can predict the chronological age with just a few hundred methylation sites. This clock is a much better predictor than biological age, and there are companies already offering tests that use this innovation.

We're also finding that epigenetic mechanisms can have protective properties. The best example is resveratrol, a polyphenol found in red wine. Resveratrol activates histone deacetylases, which are enzymes that modify a component of histone, allowing histones to wrap the DNA more tightly. So this de-acetylation regulates DNA expression in a process that erases the "scratches" that have accumulated on the CD that is our DNA. The result is that those areas are reactivated, and the genome is restored to a younger state.

And as for the other known epigenetic mechanism that appears to contribute to life span, Yousin used the lymphoblasts of our centenarians to study hundreds of miRNA and showed that the levels of many of them declined with aging. But she also found a cluster of miRNA whose levels were dramatically elevated in almost a third of the centenarians — some by as much as one hundred times the levels in other centenarians and members of the control group. She also found that some miRNA inhibit the activation of the IGF-1 receptor. Since our previous study had received criticism for the fact that our lymphoblasts might have their own problems, Yousin confirmed that the same miRNA were elevated in the centenarians' blood. So now we had yet another group with a genetic mechanism that inhibited the activation of their growth hormone pathway. Over time, we have found genetic explanations for decreased growth hormone action in more than half of our centenarians, so I've been converted — I now believe that it *is* a very important factor for exceptional longevity.

Incidentally, if you're wondering why we don't measure growth hormone levels themselves, it's because it's the wrong test. Growth hormones are secreted during the day in peaks that are hard to target unless you sample the blood every few minutes. Also, growth hormones decline with aging, and IGF-1 is secreted based on demand from tissues, not just orders from growth hormone, and that's how its levels are maintained.

Our genetic findings led Sofiya Milman, Einstein's director of human longevity studies, to wonder if people who had the lowest IGF-1 levels lived longer than those who had higher levels. To explore this question, she sent plasma samples from our centenarians to a state-of-the-art facility to measure many hormones, including IGF-1 levels. She found that twice as many of our centenarian women with the lowest median IGF-1 levels lived three years longer than those with the highest median IGF-1 levels.

This is a striking result that, combined with our genetic data, has compelling implications. Most compelling, perhaps, is that the women with the lowest IGF-1 levels had about half the mortality of the women with the highest IGF-1 levels. But Sofiya did not see the same correlation among the men. Although on average women live two to three years longer than men, nobody had looked at gender effects on aging, and it turns out that those differences are significant. In retrospect, one of geroscientists' big sins in studying the biology of aging was that our laboratory studies used mainly male rodents because we reasoned that menstrual cycles could change behaviors and metabolism in female rodents, though this argument has never been confirmed.

Sofiya also wanted to know what was happening to the cognition of the women whose IGF-1 levels were low, given that higher levels of IGF-1 are associated with better cognition, but the female centenarians in our study who had the lowest IGF-1 lived longer than the others. Surprisingly, rather than being cognitively impaired, these women had only half the impairment of those with higher IGF-1 levels. In the men, there was a tendency for an opposite effect, but we don't have enough information to draw a conclusion yet.

The last question that we wanted to

answer regarding IGF-1 was how it affects muscles. Because IGF-1 is a major growth and maintenance hormone, Sofiya wanted to know if living longer means living weaker. After testing the centenarians' muscle mass, grip strength, and walking speed, she found no difference between their results and those of people who have high IGF-1 levels. Unlike women, men's muscle function seems to be slightly better when they have higher IGF-1 levels. Our interpretation of this data is that the effect of low IGF-1 on developing and maintaining muscles during our youth is significant enough to negate the effects of low IGF-1 that would theoretically make muscles weaker.

MAKING THE MOST OF OUR FINDINGS

Our study conclusions led us to believe that a drug that blocks growth hormone action could be developed, but some studies indicated that high IGF-1 was linked to better cognitive function, which we would not want to disrupt. So with Derek Huffman, we applied for a grant to test the hypothesis that IGF-1 has beneficial effects on the brain, such as better cognition and glucose metabolism, but negative effects on the rest of the body, including higher risk of cancer.

At the same time, the pharmaceutical company Amgen was developing an antibody that works against the IGF-1 receptor as a cancer treatment. Many cancers have elevated levels of the IGF-1 receptor, which we believe helps to maintain the cancer's growth. Once the drug was developed, it was administered to patients with pancreatic cancer, but it did not appear to have clinical significance. Since it had already been developed and approved for use in humans, though, we wondered if there was a way to repurpose it with clinical significance.

Along with Frank Calzone and Pedro Beltran, then at Amgen, we created a collaboration to prove that we could extend health span and life span by targeting the IGF-1 receptor the same way it is naturally targeted in centenarians. This was the exact tool that could help prove our hypothesis that blocking IGF-1 action would extend the health span and life span of aging animals. Since the IGF-1R antibodies do not cross the blood-brain barrier, we could block IGF-1 in the body without blocking its action in the brain. We wanted to learn what would happen to mice that are treated with the antibody, whether the treatment results would be different for males and females, and whether it would affect health span and life span. Even more relevant for developing a treatment was the question of whether it would work the same way in aging mice as it did in younger mice.

To ensure the safety and efficacy of the IGF-1R antibody, Derek performed a six-month feasibility study in which aging male and female mice (eighteen months old) were given weekly injections of the antibody. No significant effects on body weight, composition, or energy balance were observed in the females. In the males, muscle mass was significantly reduced but fat was not, so there was an increase in the ratio of fat to muscle.

Derek's next step was to evaluate the antibody's blocking effects on health span. As with aging itself, females and males both demonstrated characteristic declines in endurance, strength, and motor coordination. However, the females that were treated with the antibody ran 50 percent longer on the treadmill than those that were not treated, had a twofold increase in grip strength, and improved motor coordination. In males, age-related decline in exercise tolerance was modestly blocked by the treatment, but no effect on strength was observed, and coordination was only marginally improved.

While high IGF-1 levels appear to be harmful to most of the body, they have been shown to have positive effects on the heart. Treatment with the IGF-1R antibody did not adversely affect cardiac function in females and restored their diastolic function, the main heart dysfunction that comes with aging, to more youthful levels, though it did not restore these functions in the males.

Derek also performed extensive pathologic analysis on the aging mice and noted a reduction in the growth of some tumors in females, but the presence of tumors in males tended to be increased. So low IGF-1 levels seem to be of great benefit to female mice but not so much to males.

The next question was: Do females treated with the IGF-1R antibody have increased life span in addition to clear benefits in terms of health span? To definitively determine whether we can extend late-life survival, we performed a longevity study in elderly female mice, beginning at eighteen to twenty-two months of age and proceeding until death. The mice that were given the IGF-1R antibody lived, on average, about 10 percent longer than those that were not treated. Furthermore, pathology tests performed after the mice died confirmed that deaths due to cancer, the main cause of death in mice, were significantly reduced. This study not only detected low IGF-1 levels in longevity but also provided preclinical experiments on drugs that have been in human use. And it taught us a valuable lesson — it's never too late to intervene in aging!

This also led me to think differently about the animal research studies we had been doing. We switched gears from searching for clues in lab animals to searching for clusters of mutations in humans. After that, we can design a drug for humans and test its effectiveness and safety with animals first. In using this approach, we have already created rats that have a gene we artificially introduced with the centenarian mutation of the human IGF-1R and we're following them for life to see what happens as they age. If we succeed in creating the equivalent of rat "centenarians" with improved health span and life span, this will be a new model for aging research.

GROWTH HORMONES DON'T "GROW" LIFE SPAN

Regardless of the hype, I can tell you with certainty that growth hormones do not grow your life span. And even the "benefits" of taking growth hormones are often not what they appear to be. For instance, they "melt" fat, which makes muscles look more prominent, but those muscles have not become stronger as a result of taking growth hormones, as is commonly believed. People who say that taking growth hormones makes them feel great are predominantly experiencing a placebo effect.

In a 1990 study published in *The New England Journal of Medicine,* twelve elderly men were treated with low doses of growth hormones for six months, and while it was found that they lost fat tissue, gained lean body tissue and muscle mass, and experienced improved lumbar spine density, the researchers also observed a rise in fasting glucose levels and mean systolic blood pressure. This led them to suggest that long-term use could result in such conditions as hypertension, diabetes, and edema. They also questioned whether the benefits of growth hormones were any greater than what could be achieved simply through exercise. And the study's author, Daniel Rudman, was clear about his belief that taking growth hormones has no affect on longevity. In response to the fact that manufacturers of "antiaging" products were pointing to the study as evidence of growth hormones' efficacy in their products, *The New England Journal* even went so far as to run an editorial in 2003 saying, in no uncertain terms, that that was deceptive: "If people are induced to buy a 'human growth hormone releaser' on the basis of research published in the *Journal,* they are being misled."

That said, the treatment of children of short stature with growth hormones appears to be a safe one. Considering our tall centenarians whose life spans obviously were not affected by the high levels of growth hormones they experienced during puberty, it seems unlikely that hormone treatment during this period of life will cause the aging process to speed up. Though a study conducted in France indicated that the children who had received growth hormones experienced more hypertension as adults, I have not seen evidence strong enough to conclude that it is not safe for a short period of time during puberty.

But aside from the benefits growth hormones can provide to children with deficiencies, it's low levels of growth hormones that appear to be closely linked to greater life span and health span. Even if I still had doubts about the lab studies regarding growth hormones, the data about our centenarians would have swayed me. More than half of them had mutations in the IGF receptor, microRNA, or FOXO3a, and some of them had more than one of these mutations. So the most promising longevity pathway may turn out to be treatments that lower or partially block these hormones.

FIVE:
UNRAVELING THE
LONGEVITY MYSTERY
DEEP INSIDE OUR CELLS

Spoiler Alert: Mitochondria don't just generate power

Scientists have been studying cells for more than three centuries, and we thought we had unlocked most of their mysteries or at least understood their most important functions. But about fifteen years ago, Hassy Cohen noticed something that was entirely unexpected — mitochondria, the organelles in cells that we had always thought of as energy producers, were actually doing much more. But for the revolutionary nature of that discovery to be appreciated, we need to step back and take a quick tour of the history of the cell itself.

When Robert Hooke first noticed tiny structures in a slice of cork that he had put under a magnifying lens in 1665, he thought he was looking at the building blocks of a plant, but he had actually been looking at the walls of the dead cork cells, not living cells. Regardless, the tiny structures reminded him of the small rooms that monks lived in called *cellulae,* and he named them *cells.* His description of a cell was published in *Micrographia,* but since he was not looking at live cells, his description did not encompass the nucleus or other parts of most living cells. Those were not discovered until 1674 when Antonie van Leeuwenhoek made the first actual microscope and saw spirogyra algae in a drop of water.

Over the centuries, we learned that cells make up all living things, that new cells are created when existing cells divide, and that all cells have essentially the same chemical composition. We also know that cells contain hereditary information that's transferred when they divide and that they are responsible for creating the energy that we can't live without. But the cell wasn't always so robust. In fact, its ancient ancestor was downright pathetic, and this is where the story of one of the latest discoveries about the cell actually begins.

A MATCH MADE ON EARTH

Cells have been on Earth for more than a billion years, but prehistoric cells existed in a crude form. They had a nucleus that contained genetic code in the form of DNA and RNA, and the nucleus was surrounded by the fluid known as *cytoplasm,* which was encapsulated by the cell membrane. But these cells had low energy capacity and low function compared with the powerful cells we have today. And as if being low-energy weren't enough of a challenge, the primitive cells were prone to corroding, or what we might call "rusting," thanks to oxygen in the environment. With so many challenges, the odds that these cells would amount to much were not good.

But one day, a life-changing meeting occurred. A low-energy "rust-prone" cell encountered a type of bacteria that didn't have much to brag about except that it happened to be very good at producing energy. Not only that, but the bacteria figured out how to defend against oxygen damage by utilizing it for the energetic process. Unable to resist the bacteria's allure, the cell invited it in and enveloped it, and this was the start of a beautiful relationship between cells and the bacteria named *mitochondria* — it was the definition of *symbiosis.* Because of this union, cells became powerful, terrifically versatile, and adaptable. The cell had officially beaten the odds.

Until recently, though, scientists had

downgraded mitochondria's importance and thought that the nucleus of the cell was responsible for most of the control. We thought that after mitochondria's initial contribution, its role was mainly to manufacture about a dozen proteins primarily involved in mitochondria's main function, oxidative phosphorylation — turning fuel to energy. It also looked like the cell was the dominant one in the relationship, giving the mitochondria orders by supplying a few hundred other proteins but not being particularly receptive to feedback or other controls. So how could this "marriage" last? The answer to that question was one of our biggest surprises yet — with regard not just to cells but also to longevity itself.

MITOCHONDRIA'S HIDDEN PURPOSE

While I was studying IGF-1 and growth hormone to learn more about their link with longevity, Hassy was studying their roles in prostate cancer. There are six proteins that bind to IGF-1, and each of them may have an independent role. It's a complex system, but Hassy was mainly interested in IGF-1 binding protein 3, or IGFBP3. He was using technology to "fish" for partners that bind to IGFBP3 to understand IGFBP3 binding actions and interactions, but he was running into a problem — there was a protein stuck to it that was not matched in the coding in our chromosomes.

Then he discovered that this DNA sequence of the protein was consistent with a sequence in the mitochondria. At the time, scientists knew the mitochondria codes for only thirteen large proteins, but we now know that proteins that are sometimes bound to other proteins were regarded as garbage because they didn't fit into the sequence that scientists were familiar with.

After more investigation, Hassy realized that the mitochondrial genetic code for this peptide is translated by a message from the mitochondria and that the protein is assembled in the ribosomes of the cell. Meanwhile, two other groups — one in the United States and one in Japan — had made the same discovery almost simultaneously. Because scientists had previously had no idea that mitochondria were producing peptides, this revelation about the secret life of mitochondria opened up a new field of biology that we had completely missed. As it turns out, mitochondria might be manufacturing *hundreds* of peptides! They're hiding in the mitochondrial chromosome as "genes within genes." And because we had no idea that there are genes for these proteins, they had not seemed significant enough to investigate.

The three groups all showed in a cell-based experiment that the first "new" peptide — which the Japanese group from Keio University had named *humanin* — protected neurons from the damage that can be inflicted on them when incubated with the Alzheimer's-related protein beta amyloid. Humanin, the first mitochondrial-derived peptide (MDP) that was discovered, came from the mitochondria DNA. This discovery eventually led to the discovery of hundreds of other MDPs and their roles in aging and resiliency to age-related diseases.

But at that time, we didn't know if humanin had a physiological role in animal models, so Hassy created an assay to measure humanin levels in the blood and showed that it circulates in very high physiological levels. That's when we decided to do an experiment at Einstein to try to find a role for this peptide in physiology and aging.

But what were the possibilities exactly? Well, the mitochondria could use the peptide to communicate inside the cells or with the cell's nucleus to say, in effect, that they're okay or not okay, that they're producing enough energy for the cell or that they aren't, resulting in some adaptations. But since humanin is measured in high levels in the blood, could it also be communicating with distant organs? I thought of an experiment that all of us agreed was crazy because it would skip preliminary studies, but we decided to give it a try anyway. The idea for the experiment was based on what we already knew about communication between organs. As we saw in chapter 2, leptin is produced in adipose tissue and travels in the blood to the hypothalamus area of the brain, where it inhibits hunger and glucose production, and I wondered if the mitochondria would have a way to communicate directly with the hypothalamus — the control center of energy metabolism. Maybe the mitochondria were sending messages to the hypothalamus via humanin to regulate metabolism in the entire body, not just the brain. To test this hypothesis in our lab, we infused very small amounts of humanin into the third ventricle of the brains of rats, near the hypothalamus. The result was that the hypothalamus completely took charge of metabolism — the humanin ordered the hypothalamus to improve insulin action outside the brain, and in our experiment, it accelerated the ability of insulin to shut down the production of glucose from the liver. Humanin had caused the brain to act as if we had delivered insulin near the liver to signal that the mitochondria were producing sufficient energy and that the body did not need more glucose. We had nailed our crazy hypothesis. Through MDPs, mitochondria communicate with the brain, and that is partly why the hypothalamus controls metabolism.

To confirm that the humanin infusion slowed metabolism directly through the brain, we started by confirming that humanin did not spill into the blood. Next, we noted that the central effects of humanin on insulin action in the liver were triggered by a hypothalamic messaging pathway (STAT-3). When we inhibited STAT-3, we blocked the effects of humanin. This was consistent with the fact that humanin did not have a direct effect when incubated with liver cells, again suggesting that the actions of humanin on the liver are mediated in the brain. Finally, when we provided a single treatment of humanin to a model of diabetes in Zucker rats, in few hours blood glucose dropped to nearly normal levels, suggesting it may have a role in energy and glucose metabolism and may be antidiabetic, as it inhibits glucose production in the liver.

Clearly, mitochondria are more in charge than we had realized, and that's because of MDPs. Earlier studies had indicated that mitochondrial number and function appeared to decline with aging — and that many of the age-related diseases are linked to mitochondria and their ability to function well — and in light of our own studies, it appears that MDPs may have a central role in the modulation of aging. While humanin levels decline with aging, our centenarians and their families have elevated levels. At age ninety-five, Frieda held the record for the highest humanin levels out of hundreds of people whose levels Hassy had measured. We don't know, however, if her humanin level occurred naturally or if the level was high because she needed it to protect against stress.

From the perspective of longevity, humanin was one of the most promising MDPs we had identified so far. But there was no hope in persuading investors to get behind development of a humanin drug, because Ikuo Nishimoto, the Japanese physician and pharmacologist who had secured the patent, had died and the patents he had filed for drug development had expired. When a patent expires, it's similar to when a song or a book becomes part of the public domain, and the public can use it freely, without copyright concerns. If a drug were to be developed, it could immediately be reproduced by every other pharmaceutical company, so there is currently no clear business plan for development of such a drug. Hassy kept experimenting and found that when we changed the binding site of IGFBP3 on amino acid number 6 of the humanin peptide, humanin action was improved dramatically both in cells and in brain experiments. But when we asked to secure the patent for this analog, we learned that Nishimoto had patented all the options on the humanin peptide, including the IGFBP3 binding site. So our patent application was rejected for not being original, and a drug that could be doing so much good is doomed to go undeveloped.

It's not as if biotech companies don't see the incredible promise of a humanin drug, but there's no overcoming the reality that they can't get the money to develop it when there's no patent. This fact of life is just one of a multitude of roadblocks to making effective drugs available to the public.

When Frieda moved to a continuing care community in her late eighties, she found herself surrounded by well-educated bridge players. Having had little formal education herself, she saw the pastime as a wealthy person's "entitlement" and felt a little out of place. But that didn't last long. Not one to show the status quo much respect, Frieda started a regular poker game, and it was soon drawing its own crowds. Now, with more new friends than she could count, she felt right at home.

That was Frieda in a nutshell. She lived by her own rules, as her son Jerry Rubenstein (my father-in-law) attests. "The poker games went on for years, and there was a game where she began laughing or giggling at the table and someone who was taking it too seriously criticized her for it," he says. "So she pushed her chair back and said, 'Any game I'm playing in which I can't laugh, count me out.' And she left."

Frieda, who wore high heels well into her nineties, was a wonderful model of being true to oneself. When my wife, Laura, and I were considering buying a house on Cape Cod, we were torn about taking on another big expense. Laura visited Frieda and told her about our concerns. "Never put off your dreams," Frieda said without hesitation. She died soon after, and when Laura got the news, she turned to me and said, "Get me the damn house." That changed our busy lives in a profound way, providing us a much-needed haven to escape to when necessary (which turned out to be often).

Maybe Frieda's tenacity was ultimately inspired by the hardships of her early life. She grew up in Poland in a home with a dirt floor, where she slept on two armchairs pushed together, and it was her job to run after the coal wagon as it passed and pick up the pieces that dropped, which was the family's only source of heating fuel.

When Frieda was nine, her father left to find work in America, and the rest of the family followed him to the Bronx seven years later (except for a sister who had died of malnutrition), traveling in third-class steerage across the Atlantic. From there it was the familiar immigrants' struggle to achieve the American dream, with Frieda working in the garment industry and attending high school at night. Within a few years, she met Moishe Rubenstein, who peddled fruit for a living, and they married when she was twenty-one.

They went on to have three sons during the Great Depression, but even after the economy started to bounce back after World War II, they continued to live close to the poverty line. Living in Brooklyn by now, Moishe started a wholesale fruit business that went under before long, and his next venture was an outdoor fruit stand that required him and Frieda to work long hours six days a week — no matter how fierce a winter they were experiencing — to make ends meet.

Moishe died from complications of diabetes in 1967, leaving Frieda a widow in her late fifties. She remarried a few years later, at which point life finally became less of a struggle and she could emerge from "survival mode."

The enduring result of Frieda's challenges in life was an unshakable optimism. Jerry says, "She made a lot of friends — she was very popular — and it was because of this attractive aspect of her personality, her almost unrealistic view of optimism. I mean, *I* called it unrealistic, but it was supported by her lifetime of experiences."

Hand in hand with her optimism was a refusal to take things more seriously than necessary — a refusal to take on more *stress* than necessary. In that regard, she and Jerry — both participants in our study of centenarians — were very different. "It's not that I'm not willing to be impulsive, but I tend to take a risk only when I've studied all the risks," says Jerry, who is eighty-nine. "Early in my life, some of my friends referred to me as a grim realist. And my mother once said to me, 'You know, Jerry, it's good sometimes to be foolish.' That was an important element of her existence — that she didn't want to take life, or at least *all* the elements of life, overly seriously for very long. So she always just had this power of attraction about her."

Thanks to Frieda's sunny outlook — something she shares with many of our SuperAgers — she was able to be as emotionally resilient as she was physically resilient, right up to the end. When she broke her ankle at age one hundred, she was determined to keep enjoying life and insisted on having surgery even though her doctor thought a wheelchair would be a safer option. She loved to dance, and there was no way she was willing to be confined to a wheelchair.

She was home from the hospital the day after her surgery and had a smooth recovery, and we were able to fit in a few more waltzes before her hospitalization at age 102. It was the first time she had been hospitalized for an illness, and I was there when the astonished resident discovered just how physically healthy she was.

"How many medications are you taking?" he asked her.

"I'm not taking any pills," Frieda said.

"You don't understand. I mean in the morning when you sit for breakfast, you must take some drugs?"

"I understood what you said, but I am not taking any drugs or pills."

She really was that healthy — no prescription drugs for her. But by that time, she *had* been showing signs of memory loss. When we would visit her, she was often surprised even though we had scheduled with her ahead of time. But instead of being disoriented by our "surprise" visit, when we explained things to her, she would say something to the effect of "This is so great, because I'm pleasantly surprised twice — when you call and when you arrive."

Frieda died in 2008 at age 102. One of her siblings had made it to her nineties, and her father lived to 102. And as for the good health Frieda enjoyed, beyond whatever role science has played, there's one thing that we know was *not* a factor.

"She didn't believe in exercise," Jerry says. "As she got to be quite old, people would always ask her for the secret of her longevity, and she would sarcastically say that she got a lot of exercise at the fruit stand, which had been fifty years earlier."

Jerry, on the other hand, does believe in exercise. He took up singles tennis in his midforties, playing three or four times a week, and he still plays twice a week and appears to be in great health. And based on the results of the yearly cognition test we administer as part of the Longevity Genes Project, his mind is actually becoming sharper, although he admits to a little "preparing." One of the tests asks study participants to name as many fruits and vegetables as they can in thirty seconds. His score was off the charts, and when I asked him about it, he said he had visited the grocery store the day before and memorized as much of the produce section as he could. So on that cognition test, his score was less about memory than about a determination to win, but if you're sharp enough to come up with the idea to visit the produce section before the test, you're doing fine.

And thanks to that determination, Jerry has come a long way from the poverty line he lived so close to in his youth, when he thought he would end up working for Murder Inc. Living in Brooklyn's Brownsville neighborhood, he was surrounded by organized crime, and as he watched his friends go down that road, he came to believe that that was just the way life worked. Luckily, he learned that life actually offers many other career opportunities when he attended Brooklyn Technical High School. From there, he went on to the City College of New York, taking classes at night and working for a delivery service during the day. After graduating with a degree in accounting, he was admitted to the U.S. Navy Officer Candidate

School and ended up getting an extensive tour of the Western world courtesy of the navy.

When he had served his forty months, he took a job as a chartered tax adviser but found the work unsatisfying. "My goal in life was to become independently wealthy, *independent* being the key term, and that wasn't going to happen at this middle-sized public accounting firm." So he took a job as a controller with a trucking company that offered more opportunity, and he remained in the trucking industry until the early '80s — a career during which he achieved his goal of financial independence *and* negotiated with Teamsters president Jimmy Hoffa.

"You'd tell him beforehand what it was you wanted to talk about, and by the time you got there, he knew as much about your company as you did," Jerry says of Hoffa. "And if you didn't have a sound argument, it was over."

In this case, Jerry had a sound argument. His company, which was unionized, wanted to start a new full-truckload service but couldn't afford to do it unless Hoffa granted an exception to the National Master Freight Agreement and allowed them to pay the same wages and benefits as nonunion companies were paying. He agreed, and Jerry had a successful negotiation with Jimmy Hoffa under his belt.

When Jerry got out of the business, he had enough assets that he and his wife, Bernice, could live out the rest of their lives comfortably, but when it came to leaving work behind, semiretirement was the best he could do. "I knew that boredom was a real threat to me. I knew that my mind would atrophy. What was going to challenge me? I wasn't an academic. I wasn't going to sit around reading books." His solution was to handle management for a leveraged buyout fund as a senior adviser in a half-time arrangement where he set his own hours. "I wanted to play tennis and go to the opera, and I didn't want any questions asked. Oddly enough, they agreed to it."

Around the same time, Jerry became involved in nonprofit work, most of it having to do with classical music, of which he is a great admirer. The project closest to his heart has been the Philadelphia Chamber Music Society, which he helped to found. "I'd watched all these not-for-profits go broke, and I undertook to form this society with the founder [Anthony Checchia] on the premise that we'd run it like a business." Thirty-four years later, the PCMS does sixty concerts a year, and it's never had a deficit year — even though ticket prices are about 40 percent of what they would be for a comparable show in New York City. Jerry has been as passionate about sharing the music with a wide audience as he is about the music itself.

For the past few years, Jerry has devoted much of his time to his role as Bernice's caregiver. They moved into a continuing care center after she suffered a stroke, and as his son-in-law and a scientist studying SuperAgers, it's rewarding for me to see the determination he's able to bring to his new role thanks to his good health.

Whether Jerry has inherited his mother's exceptional longevity like the offspring of many centenarians in our study have — or her high humanin levels — remains to be seen, but there's no question that he has inherited the fortitude to travel a long way. Although his journey hasn't taken him from the Old World to the New World like Frieda's, in a sense, he has come just as far.

"Several years ago, Bernice and I drove through my old Brownsville neighborhood where I was going to be a gangster," he says. "It's never been gentrified, so it still looks exactly like it did when I left it seventy years ago. We were on our way back to an apartment we had on Fifth Avenue, and I said, 'You realize it's only going to take forty minutes to drive from here to Fifth Avenue, but it took most of a lifetime to achieve it.'"

And even after all that traveling, it's clear that he's ready for more.

A CohBar Is Born

There was nothing we could do to change the patent situation with humanin, but Hassy and I decided to start our own biotech so that the next time a significant discovery was made, we could work together to test the treatment, secure the patent, and make it available to people as quickly as possible.

CohBar set out with the mission to increase healthy life span by developing treatments for the underlying metabolic dysfunction driving the diseases of aging, including NASH (nonalcoholic steatohepatitis), obesity, cancer, type 2 diabetes, fibrotic diseases in many organs, and cardiovascular and neurodegenerative diseases. In addition, we have found peptides that seem promising as anticancer therapies and antifibroptic therapies that have promising clinical targets. And since we were primarily focusing on mitochondrial-derived peptides, we wanted to come up with a clever name that incorporated or suggested mitochondria, but every one we liked had already been claimed. One potential name after another got crossed off our list, but we had to come up with something before we could register the business. Finally, on a flight from Finland, as the plane was touching down at JFK, I had an idea for a name that I was sure nobody else had claimed. I called Hassy from the runway.

"What about CohBar?"

"It sounds like a strong name," he said, "but what's the connection?"

"The connection is between *C-O-H* and *B-A-R.*"

And then it clicked for him. I still don't love it, because I prefer that the vision be part of a name, but that's the name we registered, and CohBar was born.

When we decided to form the company, we promised each other that we would not make the same mistakes that put 95 percent of biotech start-ups out of business. And while that success rate didn't sound promising, because we are both M.D.s and biologists doing a lot of lab-based research, we had a clear understanding of what we needed to do to achieve our goals. We also had the benefit of having served on the advisory boards of numerous drug companies, and we thought we knew a lot about what was involved in drug development, including the laws that govern it. So we had a solid foundation and agreed that if we did not make the mistakes that others had made, we would have a good chance of success.

Although we have kept our pledge, we didn't know that we could make plenty of our *own* mistakes that no one else had made. And we've made a lot of them. But we've come a long way from the garage in Pasadena that was our first headquarters. We had gotten off to a slow start with some executives who didn't turn out to be a good fit, but then we recruited John Amatruda, a Yale-trained endocrinologist who had been the head of Merck's diabetes franchise and developed Januvia, one of the bestselling drugs for diabetes. I was on Merck's advisory board at the time and admired John and his success in bringing the drug from preclinical testing to its status as a market blockbuster. John has become one of my best friends and a partner in various ventures, and after he retired from Merck, we invited him to join us at CohBar because he was the best person to advise us on drug development. We were committed to recruiting the very best people we could find, and while we were at it, we also invited David Sinclair, a top geroscientist who had formed several successful biotech companies, including one called Sirtris Pharmaceuticals that was eventually bought by Glaxo-SmithKline for $720 million. David is also one of my closest friends and collaborators.

By 2010, we were making headway with our research, but developing new drugs costs millions of dollars, so to accomplish our goals, we needed to find people who believed in what we were doing and were willing to invest in us, which was something neither one of us had had much experience with. Eventually, we began to meet people who were interested in investing, which was encouraging, but they didn't have the means to invest the type of money we needed.

Then one Friday afternoon, I was sitting at my desk, and I received a call from a man who spoke English with such a strong Chinese accent that I couldn't make out most of what he said. But I did hear the word *longevity,* so I asked him to write me an email. About an hour later, I received an email from him introducing me to his boss, a Mr. Liu, who he said was the biggest private owner of gas and oil concerns in China and who happened to be interested in longevity research.

And the email said one more thing: "Mr. Liu will be happy to see you on Tuesday in Beijing."

I was skeptical, to say the least. Try doing due diligence on "Mr. Liu" in China. There are millions of Mr. Lius from China on the Web. I responded politely, though, and invited Mr. Liu to meet with me Tuesday at Einstein instead, thinking that would be the end of it. A few hours later, he replied that Mr. Liu and his associates would be there on Tuesday morning. *Oh God,* I thought, *what have I gotten myself into?* Were these men wealthy businessmen or con artists?

On Tuesday morning, they arrived at Einstein in a Cadillac SUV, and it turned out that Mr. Liu didn't speak a word of English. His translator told me that many of Mr. Liu's family members were elderly and sick and that he wanted to do something to change that. In China, the problem of sickness among the elderly has an added complication because the ratio of elderly people to young people is nearing 2:1 due to the one-child policy from 1979 to 2015; if that child moves away, there is no one to care for the aging parents. The translator also said Mr. Liu was making so much money that he wanted to do something good for the world.

During his visit, I showed him our labs, and he met with other faculty members at my center and gave a presentation. And at the end of the day, we were having dinner at a Chinese restaurant in the Bronx when Mr. Liu's translator said, "I am going to invest $10 million in CohBar." Mr. Liu gave me a few minutes to regain my breath before explaining how any profit would be reinvested in CohBar. Suddenly, our dream seemed to be within reach.

It ended up taking months to do the paperwork, and on the day we were supposed to sign an agreement, our attorney, Les Fagan, was still not satisfied with the due diligence and was urging us to refrain from moving forward. Saying, "No, thank you," to a $10 million gift was not something that Hassy or I wanted to have on our records. We needed a miracle.

And we got one.

The afternoon of the meeting, Mr. Liu showed up grinning from ear to ear and holding up his phone, gesturing for us to watch a video.

I looked at Hassy. *What in the world . . .*

As everyone crowded around his screen, he pushed Play, and there he was, ringing the opening bell at the New York Stock Exchange that morning. His own company had just gone public.

Les turned to us. "Sign the agreement," he said. "That's plenty of due diligence." (We later found out that my wife's law firm was one of the firms that did the due diligence for the upcoming public offering of his company.)

A few months later, Mr. Liu sent us the first $1 million.

SEARCHING FOR PROMISING PEPTIDES

By the time we had received Mr. Liu's first installment, CohBar had identified six peptides that had similarities to humanin. Hassy's group named them *SHLPs* for *small humanin-like peptides,* and each of those peptides seemed to protect against at least one age-related disease. One of them was active against cancer, for example, some of them were active against Alzheimer's, and many had overlapping effects. And in addition to protecting against Alzheimer's, it appeared that SHLP-2 was similar to humanin in its action on metabolism. (We now know that SHLP-2 may also have protective effects against neurodegenerative diseases.) So all of a sudden, Hassy and CohBar were identifying all these other peptides that seemed to have real promise, but around the same time, the Supreme Court weighed in on the Myriad decision, which stated that naturally occurring molecules — such as genes and peptides — cannot be patented because they already exist in nature. So the way to commercialize peptides was to analog the SHLPs by making changes to them (or analoging them). This was also an opportunity to turn these peptides into drugs that are even more effective and longer lasting than the natural peptide. And by turning them into an analog, they can be patented as pharmaceuticals. We were on our way to achieving our dream to make a drug that could protect against aging itself and all the diseases associated with it!

And then the bottom fell out. A few months after we had received a total of $2.5 million from Mr. Liu, the Securities and Exchange Commission shut down his company. We learned that many Chinese business owners had started companies at the New York Stock Exchange and then taken the money back to China without following through on the business plans they had shown their investors. As it would turn out, Mr. Liu was one of the few who returned the investors' money, and the SEC eventually cleared his record, but in the process, he lost many of his businesses, and he was unable to deliver the rest of the $10 million. We felt terrible about this outcome, so we promised him that when the company begins making a profit, he will receive the first $2.5 million before we take any profit for ourselves.

The setback was heartbreaking, but one

of my best longtime friends came to our rescue. Jon Stern, the serial entrepreneur who invented the cup holders attached to seats in movie theaters and stadiums and whom we'd asked to serve as interim CEO of CohBar, introduced us to Albion Fitzgerald, who turned out to be our financial angel. With their guidance and financial support, we were quickly back in business. I had met Jon decades earlier because our parents became friends after his father had a stroke and was taken to the hospital where my father was chief of medicine. Meanwhile, Albion had made his fortune designing software and launching several technology companies, which he could have continued to do, but he decided to invest in biotech because he believed that would be more helpful to society. Ultimately, his commitment to our cause was responsible for bringing us about 75 percent of our investors.

Thanks to all that financial support, we have identified several hundred peptides and are developing new analogs. In addition to the SHLPs, Hassy has identified an exciting new peptide called *MOTS-C,* which is a promising therapy for obesity, type-2 diabetes, and NASH (nonalcoholic stentohepatitis). In addition, CohBar's science team has identified multiple other peptides that have diverse actions and potential applications for age-related diseases and are in the development pipeline.

Interestingly, people around the world have begun to identify mutations in the genetic code for the MDPs, and those mutations are associated with a variety of age-related diseases. For example, a mutation in the humanin sequence in our centenarians yields a modified version of humanin that may be involved in protection from Alzheimer's disease, a phenomenon we are studying at Hassy's lab. As discussed earlier, pharmaceutical companies require a proof of concept from a cluster of mutations in humans to justify development of new drugs, so this could prove to be an important discovery from a consumer-health standpoint as well as a scientific standpoint.

Finally, after all of this, CohBar, with headquarters in Palo Alto, has become a publicly traded company, with shares sold through NASDAQ, and a leader in the research and development of mitochondria-based therapies (MBTs) — an emerging class of drugs with the potential to treat a wide range of diseases associated with aging and metabolic dysfunction. CohBar is currently focusing on NASH with an analog to MOTS-C that is in a clinical study. Stay tuned for more good news to come as we move anticancer and antifibroptic therapy to clinical trials.

SIX:
THE QUEST TO PROVE AGING CAN BE TARGETED

As geroscientists continued researching aging and longevity, we were convinced that the biological processes that drive aging in humans could be targeted. We had already seen how knowledge about variants of CETP and APOC3 contributed to drug development. And in animal studies, we had successfully targeted common aging processes with genetic, nutritional, and pharmacologic interventions that improved health and increased longevity. These findings showed that the biological rate of aging could indeed be slowed. This alone was incredibly promising, and the skeptics who had initially rolled their eyes at our theory were starting to raise their eyebrows with interest.

Meanwhile, I couldn't help wondering if we could prevent, or at least delay, the onset of *all* the age-related diseases by targeting the primary processes that drive aging. For example, we knew that impaired metabolism was contributing to all chronic diseases and that improving it through caloric restriction in animals prolonged health span and life span. If targeting just one of the processes could do that, what would happen if we figured out how to focus on the ones that could do the most good for each individual? And what would happen if we targeted all of them?

These questions and dozens of others prompted me to collaborate with colleagues to convene a conference to determine what we could do to move toward an indication that aging deserved to be studied as if it were a disease, because without this indication, the FDA will not approve drug treatments for it. Thankfully, seven primary hallmarks of aging had already been identified by the Geroscience Interest Group, a trans-institute group in the NIH, formed by the hero of the geroscience movement — Felipe Sierra, director of the Division of the Biology of Aging at NIH. Another project that the NIH initiated is the Interventions Testing Program (ITP), designed to investigate treatments that have the potential to delay disease and extend life span. Studies conducted by the ITP confirmed that it's possible to alter several molecular and physiological processes simultaneously and that *improving one of them will frequently benefit the others.* These hallmarks of aging are fundamental to the biology of aging.

The hallmarks have evolved, and maybe more will be discovered, but each one of them is a target for aging therapy as has been demonstrated in animal models. They are also interconnected, and relieving one problem can relieve others as well. Our challenge is to find the time line for best intervention, identifying personalized therapy, and combination therapy.

Chromosome Maintenance: Damaged DNA and other cellular components can either lead to loss of cells or initiate cancers. Such damage may be initiated in part when telomeres (DNA strands at the end of chromosomes) get shorter.

Senescence: Len Hayflick has shown that there are limits to the number of times a cell can divide. When cells divide for the last time, their appearance and functions change, and these are called *senescent cells.* These cells become more plentiful with age, but there are also other reasons for senescent cells to appear. If a cell's DNA is damaged by a severe mutation, it has two choices:

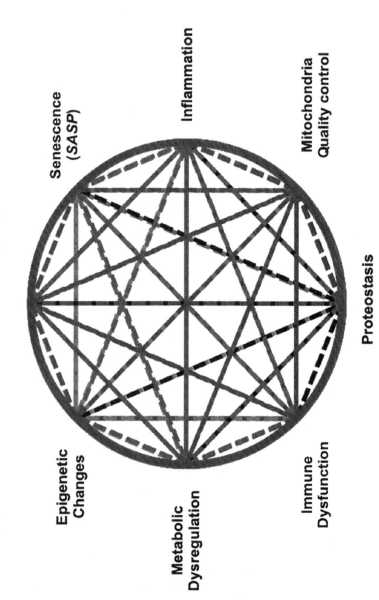

Hallmarks of Aging

- Inflammation
- Mitochondria Quality control
- Proteostasis
- Immune Dysfunction
- Metabolic Dysregulation
- Epigenetic Changes
- Senescence (SASP)

1. Commit self-destruction through a process called *apoptosis.*
2. Become a senescent cell and stop dividing.

In principle, senescence is a good thing — if the damaged cells could not become senescent, they could become cancerous, so it's a defense mechanism. But this defense does not last forever. When these "zombie" cells accumulate and are not cleared (they cannot commit suicide), they secrete inflammatory factors and other proteins known as SASP (senescence associating secretory proteins) that may change their local environment and cause cancer. So a cell could have become senescent to escape cancer, but accumulation of these cells in tissues may now actually cause it and maybe other aging diseases. *Senolytics* is the name of a group of drugs that geoscientists and biotechs are trying to develop to decrease the numbers of these cells. In preclinical rodent models, the overall health of animals with a lot of senescent cells improves significantly when they receive senolytics.

Inflammation: Inflammation is typical in aging and reflects the body's effort to repair itself when it senses breakdown. Unfortunately, this chronic inflammation is not well regulated and contributes to aging.

Mitochondria Quality Control: Mitochondria, intracellular organelles known mainly as the energy generators of cells, decrease in number, shape, and function with aging and with age-related diseases.

Proteostasis (Protein Homeostasis): The process within cells that regulates proteins' fate. Proteostasis is impaired when, for example, there is a decline in the body's ability to conduct autophagy — the process of clearing out or disassembling proteins that have misassembled in cells.

Immune Dysfunction: There is a decline in immune response against viruses, germs, and other pathogens. This increases the harmful effects of these insults, makes symptoms worse, and delays recovery. It's immune dysfunction that makes viruses like Coronavirus life-threatening to the elderly. After they have the virus for a few days their immune systems create an immunological storm that causes the clinical features that can lead to death. Rejuvenating the immune response may lower or eliminate this effect on the elderly.

Metabolic Dysregulation: Metabolism slows in conjunction with declines in the activity of hormones (such as insulin), and there are changes in cholesterol and lipid metabolism and in body fat and its distribution.

Epigenetic Changes: Several biological molecules can disrupt connections between chromosomes or disrupt the transcription from the DNA, both of which cause rapider aging. The main epigenetic players mentioned are changes in histone acetylation, DNA methylations, and microRNAs. Some of these changes are activated by interaction with the environment and can increase or decrease the activity of many genes without causing mutations. This includes stunted stem cells and regeneration. As stem cells age, they lose their capacity to regenerate new tissues.

For all hallmarks, there are mechanisms to resist and repair them that decline because of lack of adaptation to stress, which used to be a hallmark on its own. As elderly people find it harder to manage activities that had been easy for their entire lives, they experience more stress on cellular levels as well as personal levels, which accelerates most of the processes of aging.

We wanted to find an existing drug that could target many or all these hallmarks, but even if we just identified one that could target a few of them, it would be strong

215

evidence that drugs can target the roots of age-related illnesses.

We already knew that pathologies we thought were unrelated are actually so closely connected that it's impossible to disregard the integrative nature of human physiologies as we search for answers to our questions about the biology of aging. This understanding suggested that the best way to reach our goal of greater health span and life span might be with integrated approaches like developing new multi-disease preventions and therapies. For example, we have discovered that the same interventions that extend the life span of mice often improve their muscle function and heart function, reduce age-related cognitive loss, and prevent or slow the progression of several types of cancer.

It's never too late to add quality years to our lives. If we can keep our aging population healthy and active, we will prevent unnecessary suffering and offset the economic burdens of elderly people with multiple chronic diseases. By intervening early, we can minimize or avoid the damage that would otherwise be done. The ability to slow aging used to be confined to the pages of science fiction novels, but today, it has scientific credibility. The findings that show we can delay aging in mammals give us promise that we can prolong human health span, too. In fact, animal models for aging have been more representative than many models of disease because of the similarity in the biology of aging among most animals. Most animals slow down their activity and have morphological changes in their body shapes as they age and before they die. Mammalians, in particular, experience fur loss, changes in bone, muscle, and blood, and diseases specific to aging. So some of the drugs that target mechanisms of aging are effective in animals as primitive as worms and flies and as complex as monkeys.

Needless to say, everyone at the conference we'd convened had different opinions about which drug offered the most promise for our purposes, and after much discussion, we agreed to conduct a trial with the humble antidiabetes medication known as *metformin.* Generic and therefore relatively inexpensive, metformin is a biguanide, a type 2 diabetes drug that helps correct the body's faulty glucose production by improving insulin action on the liver. I was very pleased with this choice for many reasons, one of which was that I was the first researcher to describe the effects of metformin on harnessing glucose production in diabetic subjects with Ralph DeFronzo, my first mentor in the United States when I was a fellow at Yale in the late 1980s. People with type 2 diabetes who take metformin have lower glucose levels in the morning, and that influences glucose levels for the rest of the day. While we understand mechanisms that lower glucose levels, we're still investigating some of the ways that metformin targets cellular aging.

At the time of our meeting, there had been evidence that when metformin was added to the diets of nematodes and several rodent strains at various ages, it:

- delayed aging and increased health span;
- increased mean life span by an average of 7–8 percent in many studies; and
- delayed onset of diseases such as cancers in specific cancer models and functional deterioration in a model of Huntington's disease.

The ITP had also shown that mice given a combination of metformin and rapamycin, an antibiotic used to prevent organ-transplant rejection, experienced a 23 percent increase in median longevity (greater than the 10–13 percent effect of rapamycin alone for males and the 18–21 percent effect for females). While rapamycin also showed promise as a drug that might increase life span, we chose not to use it, because rapamycin's targeting abilities are still inefficient and it has major side effects in humans, including diabetes.

But the main reason I had suggested metformin for a study targeting the hallmarks of aging was because of what had been discovered in a *human* study. Researchers were given access to data from British pharmacy records that identified people with type 2 diabetes who were being treated by particular doctors as well as people who were not diabetic but were being treated by the same doctors and lived in the same general environment. The researchers showed that diabetics who were taking metformin and who were also suffering from other diseases had less mortality than members of the group who were *not* diabetic and who had less obesity and fewer diseases in general. They also had half the mortality of diabetics who were taking other diabetes medications. Specifically, the study, which included 156,000 people of about age seventy-five, found that the 78,000 taking metformin had about *17 percent less mortality* than the 78,000 people in the control group. What makes this so dramatic is that in addition to not having diabetes, the people in the control group were leaner and had fewer diseases to begin with but still had more mortality than the obese and diabetic people who were taking metformin. These observations were unanticipated and very promising.

CHOOSING AN EXISTING DRUG
TO PROVE OUR POINT

After the conference in Spain, the evidence in metformin's favor became overwhelming. In addition to the safety factor — metformin has sixty-plus years of safe use, compared with the unresolved safety issues of many other drugs that can target aging — new clinical trials reported significant reductions in the risk for type 2 diabetes, cardiovascular disease, cognitive decline, dementia, and cancer among subjects taking metformin. A randomized clinical trial known as the Diabetes Prevention Program found that metformin reduced the incidence of type 2 diabetes among more than three thousand adults by 31 percent compared with a placebo, across all ages. And the United Kingdom Prospective Diabetes Study (UKPDS) reported that metformin reduced the risk of diabetes-related death

220

among type 2 diabetics by 42 percent compared with conventional treatment.

The UKPDS also found that among subjects taking metformin, the risk of cardiovascular disease was reduced by about 20 percent, and other studies reported similar metformin-related improvements. Among them, the study "Hyperinsulinemia: The Outcome of Its Metabolic Effects" (HOME), which looked at insulin-treated patients with type 2 diabetes, found a 40 percent reduction in cardiovascular-disease outcomes when metformin was administered, compared with a placebo.

Cancer incidence and cancer-related mortality had also been shown to decline in association with metformin in several epidemiological studies. In an analysis of multiple studies of metformin's effects, cancer incidence was reduced by 31 percent, and cancer-related deaths were reduced by 34 percent. And metformin has demonstrated efficacy against breast, colon, pancreatic, prostate, liver, and lung cancers, which suggests that it works against the biology of aging itself, since that's the only risk factor these cancers share.

As for cognitive decline, cognitive performance was shown to improve among non-diabetic subjects with mild cognitive impairment (MCI) and among type 2 diabetics suffering from depression in separate clinical trials. In another study, MCI patients taking metformin showed improvement in executive functions — such as attention and memory — after just eight weeks. And observational studies reported 51 percent lower risks of cognitive impairment — with the risk being lowest among those who had been on metformin the longest — and lower rates of dementia among type 2 diabetics on metformin than among subjects on other diabetes medications.

Meanwhile, further observational studies largely confirmed what the British study comparing type 2 diabetics and nondiabetics had found: better survival rates among the diabetics on metformin than among the control group. And overall mortality was also shown to be improved when metformin regimens were begun late in life for patients with age-related diseases, such as chronic liver disease and chronic heart failure.

It's important to recognize that not all studies conducted on metformin replicate the results we have seen in many of the metformin studies, but the ones that don't are typically less rigorous. Perhaps more important, though, is that none of the studies have shown that metformin is bad for humans.

At Einstein, under the supervision of diabetologists Jill Crandall and Meredith
Hawkins, we conducted a small clinical
study — the Metformin in Longevity Study
(MILES) — of fifteen people of an average
age of seventy. For the first six weeks of the
randomized, double-blind trial, each subject
received metformin or a placebo, and then
we biopsied skeletal muscle and adipose tissues. Next, there was a two-week period of
no treatment, and then the subjects who
had received metformin for the first six
weeks were given the placebo for six weeks
and vice versa, followed by more biopsies.
And the results showed that they all had
experienced metabolic improvement. Along
with my doctoral student Ameya Kulkarni
and biologist Jessica Mar, we also studied
the biological part of the equation by
examining their tissues before and after
metformin treatment, and what we found
was that metformin significantly influenced
both metabolic and nonmetabolic pathways
inside their cells in ways that had positive
effects on some of the hallmarks of aging.
In fact, when we compared their fat and
muscle biopsies with the biopsies of young
people, the older people's pathways looked
younger.

As far as we were concerned, the case had

been made. If metformin could do all these things in studies about individual diseases, didn't it mean that it could achieve all of this by targeting aging itself? Metformin affected each of these diseases by delaying aging, so we had more evidence that aging is what's driving the diseases. If we can show that metformin will protect against a cluster of age-related diseases in humans and enhance longevity, we'll prove that the causes of aging can be targeted with safe drugs.

To be clear, it's unlikely that metformin works *directly* on all the hallmarks of aging that have so far been identified. The likelier scenario is that metformin moderately modulates the oxidative pathway of the mitochondria, which results in metabolic adaptation that causes improved insulin sensitivity and induction of autophagy. On another level, the diminished action of the mitochondria also happens to protect against oxidative stress and DNA damage, and the results reflect the fact that the cells and tissues have become biologically younger. In other words, metformin probably has a restorative effect on cells that ultimately delays the onset of these diseases and increases health span. But the important thing is that the results are the same regardless of whether the effects are direct or indirect.

So, with widespread support from biologists and gerontologists, we began to formulate a trial to prove that a drug can target the biology of aging itself: the Targeting Aging with Metformin (TAME) study.

GETTING THE FDA ON BOARD

Before designing the study, there was one crucial component of success that we needed: FDA input. If we proceeded without it, we might complete the study only to have the FDA tell us afterward that we should have done something differently and that they couldn't approve drug development based on our findings. And FDA approval is critical, because without it, a drug cannot become a standard treatment in the medical profession, and health care providers will not cover its use by patients. And, of course, if there's no demand, pharmaceutical companies will not produce the drug, and so the condition in question will not be treated with this medication despite its potentially profound benefits.

So we went to the FDA and presented our argument for a metformin trial that would test the viability of targeting aging directly. We also discussed how outcomes of the

225

studies would be consistent with our targeting of aging. And by the time the meeting was over, they'd given us their blessing to proceed.

After the meeting, Robert Temple, deputy center director for clinical science for the FDA's Center for Drug Evaluation and Research, commented for Ron Howard's *The Age of Aging,* a documentary about the science of aging: "Loss of muscle tone, dizziness, falling, dementia, loss of eyesight, all those things — to [approach] them all at once with a single treatment . . . might make a convincing case that you're doing something beyond just treating the disease. That would be something never done before. If you really are doing something to alter aging, the population of interest is *everybody.* It surely would be revolutionary if they can bring it off."

We had done it. TAME would move forward. There was one wrinkle, though — the FDA didn't want us to look at diabetes in the study.

"We don't care about preventing diabetes," one of the officials had said.

Being a diabetologist, I felt insulted. Whoever had been sitting next to me quickly grabbed my hand to signal me not to blurt out the first thought that had occurred to me. I managed to keep my mouth closed even though prevention of diabetes would have a huge health and economic impact!

Although the Diabetes Prevention Program has shown that metformin prevents diabetes, a recent effort to get an indication to use metformin to prevent diabetes in prediabetic patients with HbA1C levels above 5.8 percent was rejected. The FDA had argued that if diabetologists think HbA1C levels above 5.8 are dangerous, they should call it diabetes and prescribe accordingly. (Levels of 6.5 percent and higher are considered diabetic.)

In the case of our own study, the FDA's reasoning was that a diabetes diagnosis doesn't guarantee that everyone diagnosed will experience complications from the disease. Only 40 percent of newly diagnosed diabetics develop diabetes complications — and typically not for about ten years. The diagnosis is based on a biochemical marker that's called *hemoglobin A1C.* If you have hemoglobin A1C at about 6.5 percent, you can be diagnosed with diabetes and should get treatment to prevent complications. So demonstrating that metformin can delay the onset of diabetes complications is not as clear-cut a matter as demonstrating the delay of the onset of heart disease, Alzheimer's, or cancer. By the end of the meeting, I had a deeper appreciation for the fact that different organizations have different vantage points and agendas and that all need to be accommodated. The most important thing was that we had our go-ahead.

HOW THE TAME STUDY WORKS

Overseen by the American Federation for Aging Research (AFAR), TAME is a six-year, double-blind, placebo-controlled trial in which we have enrolled a diverse population of about three thousand adults, ages sixty-five to eighty, who do not have diabetes but who have begun to contract age-related chronic diseases or have begun to show decreased function or other markers for high risk of major age-related disease or death. People who have conditions for which metformin is currently inadvisable (such as severe kidney disease), those being treated with chemotherapy, and people who already have Alzheimer's or physical disabilities that would prevent them from attending the visits are being excluded.

Our modeling suggests that about half of adults in the study's age range meet eligibility requirements. Incidentally, although metformin may have many benefits for people younger than sixty-five, the study

228

would take longer — and cost more — if younger people were included, because it takes longer for diseases to set in at younger ages.

Our primary aim in the study is to test whether metformin delays the onset of a group of age-related chronic diseases and whether it also decreases mortality. We are looking for the initial diagnosis of a composite of major diseases of aging, including myocardial infarction, stroke, congestive heart failure requiring hospitalization, cancer (excluding prostate cancer and non-melanoma skin cancer), mild cognitive impairment, and dementia. At the FDA's suggestion, we are also assessing a broad array of characteristics that serve as a gauge of aging, such as physical functions, skin condition, hair color, and how often subjects require hospitalization.

One of the novelties of this first study of its kind is that all diseases are equally weighted when it comes to how we will analyze outcomes. Because aging increases the risk for each of the diseases in our composite, we don't know which disease will appear next for a given individual, especially when interactions between environment and genetic tendencies are considered. Research conducted by the ongoing

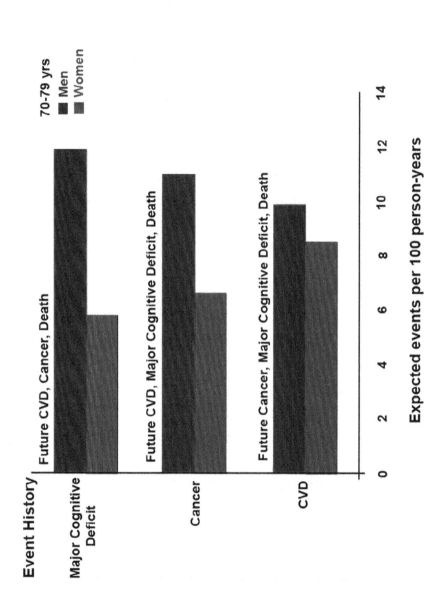

Health, Aging, and Body Composition (ABC) Study shows that when someone is diagnosed with a chronic disease between ages seventy and seventy-nine, their chances of developing another chronic disease — *any* chronic disease — is the same as their chances were for getting the first disease or any other diseases.

Let's say we follow people who have cardiovascular disease over time and determine their chances to get cancer or cognitive decline or to die. The rate is about ten events per one hundred person-years. Now, if we look at people in the same population who have cancer, their chances of developing cognitive decline or cardiovascular disease or dying is also ten. It really doesn't matter what disease you have to begin with; your chances of getting any of the other diseases is the same because aging drives them all. That's aging in a nutshell, and our hope is that by intervening with metformin after the appearance of the first disease in any given subject, we can push back the appearance of the second disease and *any* subsequent disease. Ultimately, we aim to push back aging itself.

We are also testing the hypothesis that metformin will preserve physical and cognitive function, which are obviously critical to health span. To do this, we hope to measure the time until the onset of a group of aging indicators, including major declines in cognition and mobility and severe limitations in the ability to do everyday tasks that the subjects had easily done when they were younger. And then we will see whether metformin influences the rate of decline in these areas or in slowing the decline of other quality-of-life functions. We're also collecting data on common geriatric conditions, such as fractures and pneumonia, and syndromes, such as frailty and fall-related injuries. When TAME concludes, this information will be made available to the broad research community and health care providers to guide and accelerate the pace of applied geroscience.

Although functional decline is often caused by the burden of multiple diseases, in many other cases, the decline occurs without the presence of disease, suggesting that it's simply a result of the aging process. This explanation is supported by animal studies showing that rapamycin preserves physical and cognitive function in older rodents.

The results of these studies suggest that there are functional benefits to be had by targeting aging pathways with metformin, per our hypothesis. As for gauging biological outcomes in TAME, we will test the hypothesis that metformin alters biomarkers in a manner consistent with slowed aging. Linking biomarkers to outcomes this way will allow future studies to use biomarker composites in the investigation of new age-targeting pathways and the development of new geroscience-guided therapies. We have not arrived at a consensus about a biomarker panel that would be reflective of the hallmarks of biological aging that is also feasible for a large multisite clinical trial, but we have devised a strategy to test participants on a set of blood-based biomarkers that include metformin levels, glycemic effects of metformin, and markers of clinical disease. We will conduct smaller ancillary studies to discover and evaluate new biomarkers that might be used and provide resources for ancillary studies of emerging markers and technologies for analyzing genes, proteins, and other important molecules. We are also creating a unique biorepository that will serve as a resource for identifying biomarkers that predict age-related outcomes to enhance gerontologists' understanding of metformin's aging-targeting abilities.

The protocol for the TAME study will be

1,500 mg of extended-release metformin in pill form taken once a day, and the placebo will be physically identical. We had considered using both a greater dose for greater effect and a smaller dose for safety's sake, but this is the average dose used in most clinical studies and has an excellent safety profile. Gastrointestinal symptoms like diarrhea and nausea are common but disappear in most cases after a week. Using extended-release drugs and increasing the dose weekly will also help avert side effects. There will be a three-week lead-in phase so that people with persistent GI intolerance can be removed from the study. To ensure that patients adhere to the protocol, we will use strategies that were successfully employed in the Diabetes Prevention Program, in which 75 percent adherence was achieved (several TAME investigators participated in that program). The importance of sticking to the regimen will be reinforced in phone calls and in-person visits, and subjects' pill supplies will be counted twice a year to ensure adherence.

We will conduct the study at fourteen clinical centers across the United States that were selected in a competitive review of applications, and they all have principal investigators with extensive experience with metformin and the field of aging. They are also members of the TAME steering committee and have collaborated on both the study design and the protocol. And Merck & Co. will generously provide the metformin and the placebo at no cost.

WHO'S GOING TO PAY FOR ALL OF THIS?

We had thought that designing the study would be the hardest part of the battle. Once again, we were wrong.

The problem with studying a concept that has never been studied — the problem with *innovation* — is that it's inherently risky. What if we don't prove what we set out to prove? There's always the chance of that, but even more so when what you propose really would mean a revolution in health care. That's how we lost our shot at obtaining the financial support of the National Institutes of Health, which funds biomedical and public health research for the U.S. government and which we had been counting on to cover half of our $77 million budget. There's also the fact that there's a lot of competition for funding and the NIH only has so much it can allocate, so they prioritize based on diseases that are most prevalent.

The fund-raising campaign started out wonderfully, with an extremely generous commitment from a young billionaire to fund half the study in hopes that the NIH would match his contribution. An interesting note: I had initially tried to raise funds among older people, thinking that those who best understand the decline that comes with aging would best understand our reasons for wanting to delay it, but it seemed that older people didn't believe we could truly do something about aging. While they may have had the money to help, they didn't have the hope. On the other hand, young billionaires have both. (The billionaire philanthropist who wishes to remain anonymous is in his forties.)

As for that match, although the NIH had initially expressed interest in partnering with us on the project, the reviewers ultimately turned us down for a grant — twice — ostensibly because they were not convinced that the biology of aging can be treated as a whole. And that sums up the NIH's level of risk tolerance. Obviously, the role of a medical trial — or any trial — is to make a case for a particular argument. If the judge is already convinced of the merits of the argument, there would be no need for a trial. As we have learned the hard way, governmental conservatism can be an impossible obstacle to raising funds for an innovation that promises to improve the health of a large segment of the population in a radically different way from anything else that has been attempted.

In addition to conservatism, there was the fact that the reviewers of our proposal were unfamiliar with the latest developments in geroscience, and as could be expected, politics were also involved. In the end, our expectation that we would receive the NIH grant cost us precious time that we could have spent fund-raising, and the whole process was set back by two years. Suddenly, we had to scramble to come up with $38.5 million.

Fortunately, we have AFAR as a partner. My history with AFAR goes back to 1996, when the field of aging studies was sparsely populated and the organization gave me my first grant, which allowed me to gather the data I needed to then get an NIH grant for much more. As it turned out, both grants were for similar research (I hadn't expected to get them both), so I went to AFAR and told them about something else I wanted to do: a study of centenarians. They liked the idea, and so I got my first official funding for studying centenarians. (My father-in-law had actually been the first person to provide me with funding, and I used the $25,000 that he gave me to compile the preliminary data that I presented to AFAR. Preliminary data is *very* important to getting grants.)

A few years later, AFAR began offering the Paul B. Beeson Emerging Leaders Career Development Award in Aging, which is named for the infectious diseases expert who served as Yale's chief of medicine for thirteen years. The grant is given to ten M.D.s a year with an interest in the biology of aging and, potentially, careers in gerontology. And this support of budding gerontologists has transformed the field of aging research to the point where there is a large pool of scientists with diverse areas of expertise — most of whom have received AFAR grants. For example, Dr. Ned Sharpless, who is director of the National Cancer Institute (NCI), is a Beeson scholar and has shown great interest in TAME for some time.

I serve on the AFAR board's executive committee as scientific director, so when it came time to publicize the TAME study and raise funds for it, I knew they would help. AFAR has contributed to the costs of our meetings with the FDA, members of the

U.S. Senate, and several NIH institutes, and it also organized the competitive review process for choosing the clinical centers where the study will be conducted. I couldn't have asked for a better partner or nicer, more committed people to work with, in particular Executive Director Stephanie Lederman and Deputy Director Odette van der Willik, whose vision is as expansive as mine.

And when it comes to fund-raising, you need all the help you can get. A good example of the diverse challenges of raising money for a particular piece of the health care puzzle is what happened when I requested funding from the Department of Defense, which invests significant resources into disease research. During my meeting with then Senate Appropriations chairman Thad Cochran, who's from Mississippi, I made sure to tailor my pitch to his sense of regionalism.

"You know, your state is doing really poorly," I said. "You have more strokes than anyone, you have more cardiovascular disease."

"Why is that?" he said.

"Well, there are two answers. First of all, your people take less metformin than any other state. But there's really a much more

239

important reason — your people are victims of the good food of Mississippi, this food you can't stop eating."

He burst out laughing. "That's great! I'll remember that! I'll use it! My people are the victims of the good food of Mississippi. I love it."

One of the reasons that getting funding is an uphill battle is that the Defense Department has a list of diseases it will fund research for, and while aging itself isn't represented on that list, diabetes is, and I had argued that metformin appears to treat the aging biological background that allows diabetes to set in, along with other age-related diseases. But the reviewers found this too hard to believe, and we were turned down for funding.

The fact is that taxpayer-funded aging research amounts to a small fraction of the funding for research into individual diseases, and this can be interpreted only as a sign of shortsightedness when considering the potential health care crisis posed by the increase in the elderly population that will occur in the coming decades.

What's ironic is that while some funding agencies think our research quest is a long shot, we've also been turned down for it not being high risk enough.

But when you cast a net as broad as the one we cast investors do turn up. One example occurred in Berlin, where I was speaking at the Undoing Aging conference. I was scheduled to do more interviews than I could count, and a couple of guys from the Boston Consulting Group, which matches biotechs with pharmaceutical companies, tracked me down.

"We need to talk to you," one of them said.

"You'll have to wait in line," I said, looking at my watch.

"You don't understand. We have a client who represents an interest that wants to invest a lot of money in aging research, and I think it's important that you meet him."

So I met with him and told him about TAME and connected him with AFAR. A week later, AFAR informed me that he believed in our research and wanted to contribute a significant amount to the study. Every time I hear about a new investor, it's music to my ears.

METFORMIN IS THE TOOL, NOT THE GOAL

When people hear me mention metformin, they often think I'm suggesting that it's the best way to target the causes of aging. While this is true, there's a lot more to the story.

241

The reason metformin is so important is that if our trial is successful, it will pave the way for even better drugs. The TAME study also serves as a template for a drug approval pathway that is more efficient and less expensive than the existing route of seeking approval to target one disease at a time. In other words, as biotechnology companies develop more drugs that target each of the hallmarks of aging, pharmaceuticals will be able to follow our study model and bring the drugs to market relatively quickly. This will allow us to make a difference for patients that much sooner — even for those who start them late in life.

Of course, it helps if the drug you're developing replicates genetics found in the human body. Because the drug's function in the body is already understood, safety issues are minimized, and development happens much faster. If a drug that replicates the function of the mutation in the CETP gene were successfully developed, for example, it could feasibly reach the market in ten years rather than the twenty it typically takes an experimental drug that requires years of preclinical testing.

Genetic studies will be a key to accelerating the drug development process as the world awaits medications that can extend their health span, and a perfect example of that is that metformin seems to do the same thing as the mutation we've seen in our centenarians.

And the broad approach to addressing disease modeled by the TAME study will be another key. Funded by hundreds of millions of dollars contributed by investors, many biotechnology companies are pursuing drugs to kill senescent cells, but they target only individual diseases rather than clusters. And most of the studies involved have been done on mice, with human trials only now beginning. So while the results have been promising — molecular biologist Jan van Deursen of the Mayo Clinic eliminated senescent cells from both younger and older mice, resulting in improved metabolism, cognition, and energy levels — these senolytic drugs aimed at disintegrating senescent cells have a long way to go before they can fulfill that promise. In the meantime, while we push for the paradigm shift toward expedited drug development, there's no substitute for the scientific process, and it's worth waiting for — remember the significant incidence of cancer among women who underwent hormone replacement therapy only to later learn that it was doing more harm than good. I promise that your patience will be rewarded with treatments that are even more effective than metformin at holding off the effects of aging. Metformin will likely be the first one available, but it will be replaced with a next generation of treatments that may incorporate metformin in combination with other drugs and will have much more powerful effects. And with the precedent established by the TAME study, those treatments will become available sooner rather than later.

SEVEN:
MAKING EIGHTY THE NEW SIXTY

For the first time ever, there are more people on earth who are older than sixty-five than people who are younger than five. And by 2050, the number of people age eighty and older is predicted to skyrocket from the 125 million estimated in 2018 to 434 million. This shift will have dire effects unless most of those 434 million people are physically and mentally healthy. China has already felt the effects of the shift in the ratio of young to old, as many elderly couples have only one child to care for them as they age. With a safety net that small, there is a significant chance that public systems will have to shoulder some of the cost of their care. And Japan may be setting itself up for the same problem, considering that deaths have been outpacing births there for the past several years, possibly in response to declining economic opportunities, and it already has the world's highest life expectancy — eighty-four — and oldest population, with 26.7 percent age sixty-five or older. Singapore's population also has a very high life expectancy, at nearly eighty-three, and that's why I am consulting for Prime Minister Lee Hsien Loong's office. To give you an idea how desperate the government is to head off a crisis, one of the questions that officials asked me is whether metformin should be put in the water supply. (My answer was *no,* of course.) I am also a visiting professor in Singapore and have been working closely with Chong Yap Seng, the obstetrician who realized that the intrauterine environment can affect rates of aging, and this is yet another reason aging should be targeted.

Those of us conducting longevity research are not the only ones racing to avert a looming world crisis. The health care industry, human service organizations, and governments are also looking for strategies to deal with this change because the costs of chronic disease and long-term care can cripple economies and lower the quality of life for many people worldwide, particularly in industrialized countries.

The need to intervene is especially urgent because health span is not keeping up with rising life expectancy. Our current approach to treating age-related diseases can delay mortality, but it does not prevent or reverse the decline in overall health, so people are sick during the last five to eight years of their lives on average and often struggle with multiple chronic diseases. The number of elderly being treated for three or more age-related diseases is increasing, and each disease requires different treatments that have the potential for adverse side effects and drug interactions. And this reality is the reason I sometimes hear groans when I tell audiences that we are looking for ways to add decades to the current life span. Nobody wants to live to be one hundred if they are going to be sick for the last forty years.

According to the World Health Organization (WHO), the increase in the aging population is predicted to be accompanied by an increase in obesity, diabetes, dementia, cancer, and the frequency of falls. Making matters worse, managing patient care for people who have three or more chronic diseases is complex and challenging. Currently, about 50 percent of Americans from ages fifty to seventy-four suffer from impaired mobility, about 33 percent have hypertension, more than 10 percent have heart disease or diabetes, and many have more than one of these conditions.

So that patients receive adequate case management, the health care system will need to create and implement multidisciplinary approaches. And while leaders in the health care industry understand that preventive care is better than reactive care for people and for the economy, it will not be enough to turn the tide. But the drugs for targeting aging that are already in development can do just that, and in the process, they can also forever change the way we think of aging. Maybe most important, they can help us to head off the problems that would otherwise accompany the dramatic rise in the aging world population that many predict.

Imagine a world where not only the wealthy have access to the best health care and are therefore most likely to live long, full lives. Currently, longevity is largely a matter of education and socioeconomics, and it's a problem that will adversely affect more and more people if it's not corrected. In the United States, the opioid epidemic and the obesity epidemic played a leading role in the nation's first decline in average life expectancy (by a tenth of a year) in more than fifty years, and the populations in the poorest, least educated areas live a full ten years less than the average. So in addition to becoming poorer, the poor are becoming shorter-lived. But imagine a world where rich and poor have the same access to inexpensive longevity drugs — ones that cost a tiny fraction of the cost of treating an individual disease. The bad news is that the gap won't close quickly. Developing just one new drug can cost a billion dollars or more and 95 percent of efforts fail, so the first geroprotective drugs will probably be very expensive when they are first introduced. But, the good news is that Metformin is one of the least expensive drugs on the market, and once it's approved as a geroprotective drug many people will be able to afford this option. The other good news is that the prices of the new drugs will go down as the need for them increases. Several years ago, University of Southern California economist Dana Goldman and AFAR board member Jay Olshansky estimated that the financial benefits of commonly prescribed age-delaying drugs would amount to $7 trillion in the United States by the year 2050. Imagine how much faster scientific advances — in *all* areas of science — could be made if those trillions of dollars were not tied up in the treatment of the individual diseases of aging. And imagine the contributions to society that people could make when they are mentally and physically healthy enough to work and volunteer into their eighties and nineties. Some people argue that we don't need more "old people," but in many countries people age sixty-five and older contribute more than 40 percent of the economy. They have worked and saved, their children have left home, and they have more resources and spend more money than younger people. In fact, if everyone age sixty-five and over were to suddenly die, the economies around the world would collapse.

When I opened a panel on aging in Davos, panel members pointed to investments in technologies that will make life easier for the elderly, from phones with bigger screens and buttons to household robots, suggesting that this is how the economy will grow and be sustained in the face of lower birthrates, which means less income to support health and human services for older people and fewer people to care for them. But when I ask older people what's on their wish list, at the very top is getting a job. Whether they need the income or not, they want to be involved and contribute in whatever way they can. For all those reasons, improving health span is desperately needed. When he was ninety, then Israeli president Shimon

Peres told me that as long as he had more plans than achievements, he wasn't ready to stop. Amazing, considering his wealth of achievements.

Unfortunately, one of the biggest obstacles to entering this new frontier in health span and longevity is the myth that there is nothing we can do about aging; it cannot be targeted. It can be. And our goal is not just to delay aging and possibly stop it but also to reverse its negative effects. When I attended the conference "The Progress of Regenerative Medicine and Its Cultural Impact" in 2015 at the Vatican, Vice President Joe Biden spoke about how complicated it is to treat cancer, and when Pope Francis took the podium later, he said, "I still hope that there will be a simple drug and a cheap drug that will treat cancer for everyone who gets it around the world." And when it was my turn to speak, I told them about metformin. "Well, I don't have this medicine," I said, "but I have a medicine that prevents cancer, and it is very cheap medicine. And it happens to prevent not only cancer but cardiovascular disease and Alzheimer's and mortality." As we discussed in chapter 6, medications such as metformin are being used by humans and showing astonishing positive side effects, and in the near future, we will have new drugs and combinations of drugs to target the hallmarks of aging that will work significantly better. So if we can target aging effectively now, why not *do it* now instead of waiting for the inevitable crises to occur? In terms of the cost to society, this approach is extremely affordable. In 2005, Goldman and colleagues at the RAND Corporation calculated the cost to society of various treatments to extend a human life by a year, and the cost of a geroprotective compound that would extend health span by ten years came in at the rock-bottom cost of $8,790, compared with cancer treatment at $498,809 and a pacemaker at $1.4 million. Isn't this an offer that we as a society can't afford to refuse?

The healthy longer lives that the Super-Agers in the Einstein studies enjoy allow them to pursue new opportunities and ventures, help raise their grandchildren, and provide rich benefits to the world at large because of their wisdom and life experience. Imagine a world where this is the norm for everyone. The only thing standing between that reality and the one we have is money.

THE PRICE OF PROGRESS

The road to drug development is an expensive one involving multiple phases of clinical research, formation of a biotechnology company, and, hopefully, sale of the drug to a pharmaceutical company that can finance phase-two and phase-three trials, in which effects of a drug are tested on as many as three thousand volunteers, usually across many sites, sometimes around the world — a process that costs tens of millions of dollars. Because the results of animal studies are insufficient to know how a drug will affect humans, a biotech needs to create a drug for testing in humans. The drug must be based on analogs since natural systems and organisms themselves cannot be patented, but even if they *could* be patented, analogs' modified versions have greater efficacy and a longer half-life than the natural ones.

Once the analogs have been created and the patents have been acquired, it's time for the phase-one study, in which healthy volunteers are administered increasing doses of the drug to test its safety and its pharmacodynamics — its general effects on the body. If problems are encountered, the formula may need to be diluted, the dosage may need to be adjusted, or any number of other adjustments may need to be made to establish the drug's safety. In phase two, doses that are hypothesized to be therapeutic are administered to people who have the condition that is being targeted, and the drug's efficacy and side effects are monitored. If phase two establishes that the drug produces the desired effect — a finding known as *proof of principle* — it moves on to phase three to determine *how* effective it is in a population that needs the drug. But developing a drug to target age-related diseases as a group is more complicated because the FDA will not approve such a drug until it has been proved that aging *can* be targeted. Therefore, pharmaceutical companies will not be willing to foot the bill for phase three — which, in our case, would total $77 million. That's why there's so much at stake with the TAME study. And even after all the trials, only about 5 percent of registered biotechs succeed in getting new drugs to the market. It's a risky business, and that's why the future of targeting aging lies in collaboration.

COLLABORATION IS
THE KEY TO SPEED

A cooperative approach gives us a much better chance of heading off the looming health care crisis, so when I was asked to join an innovative new collaborative company as the chief medical consultant, I said yes without having to think twice. I should add that one of the reasons I didn't hesitate to join Life Biosciences is that I already knew the founders, David Sinclair and Tristan Edwards. The goal of this first-of-its-kind venture is the nurturing of individual daughter biotechs all focused on targeting different hallmarks of aging and developing drugs that will eventually prevent diseases of aging. This didn't surprise me because Tristan and David are known for their innovation and achievement in their respective fields of funding and science.

When the two founders joined forces, it was another great opportunity for me to collaborate in efforts to accelerate the targeting of aging. My primary roles are helping to ascertain whether new science findings are increasing longevity and, if so, to help to determine what indication of need we can prove relatively quickly to raise the funding for drug development and clinical studies. Essentially, we are looking for a pathway that targets aging in animals and leads to improved health and life spans. But to be ready to start creating new age-targeting drugs as soon as we get the TAME

255

results, we need to discover age-related indications *now.* And those indications need to be promising enough for pharmaceutical companies to partner with us or buy daughter companies from us as we move from the phase-one trial to phase two.

One of the things that set Life Biosciences apart from other companies is that we want everyone to be fairly rewarded. The standard practice for drug development companies is to sideline the founding academic scientists because they don't understand this totally different profession of creating a drug, protecting intellectual property, and doing safety and toxicology studies and clinical testing. While academic scientists can consult on mechanisms related to the development of specific drugs, a common complaint is that they're not always involved in the entire process and therefore are not compensated as well as they might prefer. But at Life Biosciences, we believe that there are dozens of good reasons to keep scientists fully involved for the duration of a project, including the fact that they can offer centralized advice to the daughter companies, test options in our labs or their own labs, reproduce models, and monitor and weigh in on progress, which all increase the chances of creating safe and effective age-targeting drugs in the near future. The scientists have also made observations and offered insights that can give drug development an edge. For example, we realized that if we were going to get reliable results about the biology of aging from our research animals, they had to be old. Most research is done with young animals, and their biology is so different that drugs developed for achieving something in young animals can produce very different results in older animals and ultimately fail.

I had often questioned the validity of lab experiments that used young rather than elderly animals for testing treatments to counteract the hallmarks of aging, given that the biology of aging is very different from the biology of puberty and prepuberty. Using elderly mice or rats improves our chances of achieving results that may be useful for elderly people. Life Biosciences requires that we use older animals to test if drugs designed to keep age-related diseases and morbidity at bay are effective.

Finally, after going through the birth stages of Life Biosciences, we recruited Mehmood Khan, a dream CEO who had been the vice chair of PepsiCo, and his experience and network have been extraordinarily helpful in guiding our success.

Mehmood, whom I've had the pleasure to know for many years, is also an endocrinologist who was trained at the Mayo Clinic, where we first met. He was working in the pharmaceutical industry before being hired as the vice chair of Pepsi, and he's also the one who invited me to join the company's scientific advisory board.

LONG, HEALTHY LIFE SPAN VERSUS IMMORTALITY

When Bill Nye "the Science Guy" asked me if I would want to have my brain cryogenically frozen contingent on the promise of immortality in the future, I told him that the only brain freeze I'm interested in is the one I get from Häagen-Dazs Vanilla Swiss Almond.

When I'm interviewed about the work I'm doing, people often ask if I would want to live forever. I'm not sure why the promise of being healthy until we're one hundred and then dying in our sleep elicits this question, but it does. So to be clear, while there are scientists exploring immortality — and who can say whether they can achieve this goal or whether they should? — that is not what most leaders in the health span field are pursuing. The treatments that CohBar and Life Biosciences are pioneering and those I am aware of at companies like Juvenescence and Unity are designed primarily to increase health span by many years. My hope is that we can continue to increase complementary coordination among geroscientists to keep our efforts from being siloed and move us from discovery to implementation faster.

That's exactly what we're doing at Life Biosciences. Our daughter companies are developing drugs to individually target the hallmarks of aging and develop affordable treatments. Life Biosciences provides the necessary capital and management infrastructure, makes research facilities available through its central laboratory in Cambridge, Massachusetts, and coordinates the sharing of knowledge across the organization. All founded by leading scientists from around the world, the daughter companies include:

- **Selphagy Therapeutics.** Cofounded by Ana Maria Cuervo, codirector of the Einstein's Institute for Aging Research, member of the National Academy of Sciences, and one of my most admired collaborators, and Evris Gavathiotis, a biochemist at Einstein, Selphagy is developing drugs to restore the body's ability to conduct autophagy, or clear "junk" proteins from cells. Its aim is to target aging and diseases like Alzheimer's, Parkinson's, and some eye diseases.

- **Continuum Biosciences.** Cofounded by Kyle Hoehn, a biochemist and cell biologist from the University of New South Wales, and Webster Santos, a chemist at Virginia Tech, Continuum has discovered new molecules that increase the energy that the body expends by activating the work of the mitochondria. The Continuum team is working to refine the molecules' safety and effectiveness at improving metabolism for humans, and they have the potential to treat obesity, liver disease, diabetes, and other diseases that result from storage of excessive amounts of nutrients.

- **Iduna.** Iduna is developing a way to rejuvenate cells by erasing their age and reprogramming them. It's based on the work of Shinya Yamanaka, the Japanese researcher who won the Nobel Prize for his discovery that mature cells can be converted to committed stem cells — committed to particular pathways of differentiation. In other words, they can become neurons or liver cells or any kind of cell you wish to establish. Later, David Sinclair inserted a virus to change the epigenetic landscape so that the cells lose the aging hallmark. An initial experiment showed that he could reverse glaucoma and return sight to a crushed optic nerve. Iduna will initially develop this approach for treatment of age-related diseases and ultimately for treatment of all aging cells.

The daughter companies all work independently in locations including Massachusetts, New York, Virginia, and Australia, but they also work collaboratively, and considering that in the near future we will probably need combination drugs that are developed by multiple companies, it's fortunate that the apparatus is already in place.

And indeed, there is already some great collaboration happening outside of Life Biosciences, too. For example, Unity president Nat David, scientific founder Judy Campisi, and other academicians are directing research on treatments that kill zombie cells before they can turn into cancer. Life Biosciences is also working on targeting those cells with drugs, but it is not a competition in the traditional sense. We are all working toward a paradigm in which the availability of many drugs will lead to more personalized options for treatment of diseases.

Meanwhile, when the founders of Juvenescence came to me about a new project, we were not able to get involved because the work was too similar to what we were already working on, so I shared their idea with my friend Jim Mellon, a visionary who's often referred to as the Warren Buffett of England and who has personally invested in longevity research and recruited investors to support biotechs that are working on drugs and treatments that target the hallmarks of aging. "It would be a good company. Somebody should do it," I told him, and he ended up cofounding Juvenescence in 2016. Jim is one of this movement's biggest supporters, and in addition to having become good friends, we collaborate on opportunities to educate the public and governments about the coming health span revolution.

I'm for the acceleration of the field. It just makes sense. And one of the benefits of Juvenescence's entry into the field is that it spreads the risk. At one point, Life Biosciences and Juvenescence were raising funds in Australia simultaneously, and many investors invested in both, seeing it as a way to hedge their bets. Of course, Life Biosciences would have liked to walk away with the whole pot, but the fact is that there might not have been *any* money if investors hadn't had the opportunity to lessen their risk. In fact, we are envisioning even more collaboration and possibly even merging the companies.

Another effort to share resources and accelerate the learning curve was the formation of the Academy of Health & Lifespan Research in 2019. David Sinclair and I joined with seventeen other gerontologists to found a nonprofit organization with the goal to share new longevity research at conferences, public forums, and governmental meetings through the publication of white papers. With David Setboun as president, the academy's hope is that in addition to accelerating the pace of discoveries related to health span, our efforts will result in increased public and private investment in longevity research around the world.

It's this type of research and data that encourages investors like Sami Sagol, an Israeli billionaire, to put their resources behind longevity research. Sami has interviewed almost every high-profile scientist in the world and understands that aging is a flexible condition that can be modulated *now.* He has contributed funds to research on the aging of the brain and the metabolism and the use of artificial intelligence to help solve some of the biological problems of aging. I could have asked him to support my lab or my biotech, but I decided on the spot to simply be his adviser so I wouldn't mix my own wishes with those of a man who can change the big picture. I learn something every time I'm with him at symposiums or other meetings, and he insists on staying in the same nearby hotels I do no matter how low on frills they are — he doesn't want to waste time on traveling to the meetings and doesn't require the ultimate in comfort when something that can change the world is at stake. He's an enhancer of aging research and a beautiful example of the type of collaboration required to accelerate treatments for expanding health span.

Finally, I am also helping to set up collaborations between medicinal chemists and an academic investigator aimed at designing and developing a drug and obtaining a proof of concept for its action within academia. This collaboration will help to enhance the visibility of the biotech field, encourage potential biotech investors to do the proper

due diligence, and ultimately inspire investment in promising biotechs.

THE GAP BETWEEN MAKING DRUGS AND MAKING DRUGS AVAILABLE

Ideally, all longevity scientists are looking
for innovations to speed up our ability to
identify indications, complete the necessary
research, and begin phase-one and phase-
two clinical trials. But none of that work
will lead to actual drug development without large sums of money, so scientists need
investors with big visions as much as the
investors need us. And while scientists and
visionaries sometimes view situations and
opportunities from very different angles, the
successful symbiotic marriage of the cell
and the mitochondria has set a good example for us. As a result, everyone at Life Biosciences is excited about discovering a new
frontier that can begin changing the way we
age within years. The more of these types of
collaborative companies that are created,
the faster we can realize a promising future.

Although serving as a scientific adviser to
drug development companies had cured any
naiveté that I had about how long it takes
to get new drugs to the market, until a few
years ago, I had no idea that so many factors could stop development before it even

265

started. For example, potential investors' assessment of the company's value can mean the difference between life and death for the project. In general, investors are looking for the greatest gain in the shortest amount of time and for projects with a history of success, so while a company's vision can add a lot to the value, it is often not enough to overcome an evaluator's bias that has been created by past failures. In the case of a drug that targets aging, the valuation may start high because investors are drawn to the novelty and the promise, but if we say, for example, that it will prevent aging and Alzheimer's and delay death but there is no successful track record to point to — aging is not a thing yet — the valuation will drop. So the valuation ultimately reflects a balance between the promise and past success. Therefore, any of the biotechs can run out of money anytime and fold.

For that reason, companies that are working on aging treatments need investors who believe in the science that supports these efforts even when the valuations are not great. And they need to see the potential in something that has not been done before, something on the level of a Google or an Amazon or the Wright brothers' first flying machine. We have a picture of the Wright brothers' first plane on the screens of every computer in our Life Biosciences offices to remind everyone that those who make the biggest advancements are rarely supported in the beginning. When the Wrights offered their invention to the government — at no cost — they received a form letter to the effect that theirs was just another experiment in mechanical flight that had not demonstrated a practical use and did not qualify for government support (which they hadn't asked for). Thinking about that today, our response is likely to be *Are you kidding?* So this is the story we tell other scientists and potential investors when we share our vision. We need a longer runway to get our plane off the ground, but make no mistake — we will fly.

As Bill Gates said, we overestimate the progress that will be made in the next two years and underestimate the progress we will make in ten years. Hang in there — help is on the way.

EIGHT:
STOP THE CLOCK

Our maximum potential life span as a species is thought to be about 115 years, but many people die before the age of 80 after suffering from an average of three diseases. So we have 35 extra years that we can realize, like some of our centenarians have, and we are beginning to understand how to scientifically capture those years and make them healthy. I'm on a mission to make this happen as soon as possible, and my hope is that this book will encourage people of all ages to support this mission, along with many more researchers and investors. Ideally, we can lengthen life span and also shorten the amount of time that people are sick at the end of their lives. The Centers for Disease Control and Prevention confirmed our findings when they compared the medical costs of the last two years of life for people who die after the age of one hundred with the costs for people who die around age seventy. The centenarians' costs were a third of the costs for those who died younger. This is good for individuals, families, and entire countries, and in the United States, it can help to significantly lower medical costs as discussed in chapter 7. We are ushering in a future where the norm will be for people to be healthy, active, and mentally sharp during the last quarter of their lives. And fortunately, there's no need to wait for the new drugs — there are many things you can do right now to slow the aging process and stay healthy, strong, and sharp.

But before we get into recommendations, let me explain my thinking and my limitations. First, the only recommendations that I can safely make are based on data that is derived from clinical controlled studies. The reason these are the only studies I totally trust is because the relationship between the mind and the body affects our health and can also affect the outcome of association studies. When the participants in an association study experience improvements, we don't know whether it's because of the treatment, because of something else they're doing, or because of the placebo effect. We've learned that when someone takes a drug or undergoes a treatment that they believe can help them, they are up to 40 percent likelier to show some improvements. So the mind can work for us, but it can also work against us because people who are depressed tend to die earlier than people who aren't, and there's biology behind that. Endorphins, proteins, and many other substances that are being secreted from the body and the brain affect our physical and mental health.

With clinical studies, researchers must be able to demonstrate that the intervention being used produces a statistically significant effect. But there aren't many clinical trials about longevity and the relationship to death as an end point of aging that involve human participants. So I'm also including results from some credible association studies, but not as recommendations — simply as information. It's important for me to make this distinction because the first rule we learn in medical school is "First, do no harm," or in Latin, *Primum non nocere.* So when we conduct a controlled clinical trial, we are not just looking for potential improvements — we are also looking at the side effects. In other words, what are we giving up for whatever we're gaining? In addition to that, we have established that what's good for one person can be bad for another, not just because of gender and age differences but also because of simple case-by-case differences — we're all biologically unique. But there is information that comes out of well-done association studies that can be useful, and I believe there are things that affect our health and longevity that we can't yet measure, so the jury is still out on many of the innovative ideas being tested. But when I hear stories about people taking treatments, drugs, or botanicals that have not been proved to be safe in clinical trials, I am dismayed by the lack of judgment. Even seemingly innocuous supplements can interact with medications in deleterious ways.

HOW OLD IS OLD?
Biological Versus Chronological Age

When we medical residents followed Dr. Bar Hama on rounds, he routinely asked us if we thought the patient looked older or younger than his or her age. We quickly realized that biological age and chronological age are not the same. But the impact of this realization didn't hit home for me until I watched my mother appear to age twenty years over the span of just one. When she was fifty-five, she was diagnosed with acute hemorrhagic pancreatitis and spent three months in the intensive care unit. I was thirty-four at the time, and many nights as I sat by her bed, I was afraid she would die. Her pulse was weak, she had almost no blood pressure, and her oxygen levels were barely detectable. She underwent several surgeries, including the removal of parts of her pancreas and a colostomy. While the colostomy was reversed a year later and she was able to return home, she was more like a seventy-year-old woman than a woman in her late fifties. As a Holocaust survivor, though, she was strong and motivated, and she managed to live to seventy-eight. But the last two decades of her life were wrought with medical problems and her quality of life was not good, even though we all did everything we could for her. For me, this experience drove home the critical importance of extending health span along with life span. And it also exemplified that chronological age and biological age are often not in sync.

To assess people based on biological age, scientists have been trying to agree on a standardized set of aging biomarkers. We've done all sorts of tests, from functional — can he get up out of the chair without using his hands and arms? — to biological — what's his HDL, and how long are his telomeres? — but nothing has proved to be an accurate marker for everyone. We're finally making some headway, though, as a result of getting large amounts of data and using augmented intelligence.

The FDA supports this move because bio-markers will allow us to treat people based on their biological age instead of their chronological age. This could mean, for example, that if your age is fifty but your biomarkers show that you're biologically closer to forty-five, you could wait five more years before having your first colonoscopy. The biomarkers will help us to deliver better health care because we will have better ways to predict who is at risk now and who will be at risk later.

Adding to this challenge is that we gero-scientists want to find biomarkers that we can change by interfering with the hallmarks of aging. For example, if we administer a new drug or treatment, we want to see that the person's biological age becomes younger as a result, and this is a tall order. For now, it seems that the best biomarker we have for differentiating between biological and chronological age is the mechanism called *methylation.* Interaction between the environment and the genome — epigenetics — causes changes in methylation across our genome, which modulates the activity of genes. My friends Steve Horvath and Morgan Levine, scientists at UCLA, measured several hundred methylation sites across the genome, and they are determining chronological age from a blood test. On a population level, what we see in the blood is the same as what we see in the organs. But for individuals, it may be that the biological age of one organ is different from the age of another — the biological age of your heart may be different from the age of your liver. If your heart is older, you may get cardiovascular disease. If your liver is older, you may get liver disease. And for the sake of showing how complex all of this is, adult women's breasts are biologically ten years older than the rest of their bodies' biological ages because of methylation.

Steve and Morgan also created a way to use artificial intelligence to measure our "clock," which estimates how many years people will live on average. My problem with this is that the measurement is based on the changes in methylation — and methylation may not be such a reversible process. If we give someone a drug that slows aging, the methylation that already exists may not go away. So while this test opens some interesting inquiries, I believe we will eventually come up with better biomarkers to guide us with treatment options. (More about the clock in chapter 9.)

USE IT OR LOSE IT
Exercise Promotes Health Span and Life Span

Hands down, the most important intervention we have for aging is physical exercise, which has positive benefits for males and females at every stage of life. Not only does physical activity improve our cardiovascular health, help to regulate our weight, and lower our risk of type 2 diabetes, it may also help to prevent strokes, dementia, and even cancer. Based on the existing evidence, it appears that we're meant to be physically active throughout our lives, but at some point between ages sixty and eighty, we start to lose energy and muscle strength as the biology of aging affects our whole bodies. Cardiovascular ability also declines with age, so strength training and cardiovascular exercises are particularly important as we get older. The key is to try a wide variety of activities and exercises that increase strength and bolster your cardiovascular system and to stick with the ones you like most. There's a lot of truth to the adage "Use it or lose it," and it has to do with more than just staying in shape. It turns out that aerobic exercise also provides some amazing cognitive benefits. (More about that below.)

As we age, it's also important to retain flexibility by stretching and doing practices like yoga and tai chi that help to maintain balance. My sister Osnat, who is a super trainer with studios around the world, convinced me that flexibility is important throughout life, but even more so as we age. I took her advice and believe it prevented me from having a disability. Flexibility and a good sense of balance can also help to prevent injuries. I stretch for fifteen minutes at least once a week and more often when I can. It's never too late to start exercising, but it's imperative that you start slowly if exercise is not already part of your lifestyle. Start by getting clearance from your doctor for the specific exercises you plan to do, and begin by working out at 60 percent of your capacity and slowly building up from there.

As for how much you should exercise, the answer is that we don't know yet. Just as with caloric restriction, where restricting some calories extends our life span but restricting all calories would kill us, we need to strive to find the optimal ranges for what we're trying to achieve. The type and amount of exercise that's best for you may be harmful for someone else; we're all different. We usually recommend that elderly people exercise for at least twenty-five minutes from three to five times a week. There's nothing that supports this absolutely, and there's nothing that disputes it — it's just a reasonable recommendation for the elderly population in general. When it comes to individuals, we might ask some of them to exercise more often or for longer periods of time.

While the specifics are far from clear, we know that physical activity is crucial to health span and will increase your chances of passing age eighty. The benefits of exercise for both the young and the old are greater than the benefits we have seen from any particular diet.

A study that followed more than 650,000 people over about ten years reported that moderate exercise such as brisk walking for seventy-five minutes a week added almost two years to people's life expectancy. People who averaged two and a half to five hours of exercise a week gained three and a half years in life expectancy, and people who exercised an hour a day added four and a half years. That said, keep in mind that this is an observational or association study. Maybe the participants who exercised were aging slowly and that's why they were *able* to exercise. Maybe healthy diets or a supplement regimen are the reasons for some people's longevity. Thus, while my belief in exercise is strong, as a scientist, I can't tell you that the longevity differences reported in this study were absolutely a result of exercise. But I can tell you that I exercise every day. And on days when I'm visiting my sister Netta, I exercise more because I can't resist her delicious cooking.

There was also a study funded by NIH that concluded that mortality rates for older women (average age seventy-two) who walked about 4,400 steps a day were significantly lower than the rates for those who walked about 2,700 steps a day. Mortality rates dropped even further for the women who averaged more than 4,400 steps a day and leveled off at around 7,500 steps a day. There's a commonly held belief that 10,000 steps a day is the magic number for staying healthy, but I have to tell you there isn't much scientific evidence to back that up. And if it does turn out to be the right number for people who are young or middle-aged, that doesn't mean it might not be too much for some older people.

By the way, how many steps it takes you to walk a mile depends on the length of your stride, and that length tends to decrease with age. But for the sake of calculating, if your stride is a little longer than two feet, it will take a little more than two thousand steps to walk one mile. If you're active with everyday activities on a regular basis, it's possible that adding just one mile to your day could be enough to extend your life span and health span.

The interesting thing about exercise is that, in theory, it should be bad for us. It induces oxidative stress, which appears to contribute to aging and disease, and it increases the breakdown of muscle tissue as well as causing some inflammation. And yet exercising is good for us at every age. So what's going on?

ANTIOXIDANTS AND HORMESIS

Regular exercise appears to have a positive effect on all the hallmarks of aging, and that may be due in part to a process called *hormesis,* by which a certain amount of stress can be helpful and protective because it activates many of our natural defenses. Since moderate exercise increases our metabolic rate, it leads to more oxygen free radicals in our cells. We used to think that these free radicals were strictly harmful. But we've learned that they have complex effects, some of which are helpful. For example, free radicals notify cells when they're in danger of being seriously damaged so the cells can turn up their internal antioxidant defenses.

So hormesis, the body's process of up-regulating mechanisms that protect it against oxidative stress, can be thought of as a resilience builder — you build resilience to something toxic by exposing yourself to it. Exposing yourself to the short bursts of oxidative stress that come with exercise builds your defenses against stress in general, and that slows the aging process. Exercise stimulates an enzyme called *AMP kinase* that helps maintain cellular-energy homeostasis and control lipid metabolism. Exercise also activates the nutrient-sensing protein mTOR, which works against longevity, but the benefits of exercise still by far outweigh the drawbacks.

In addition to hormesis, regular exercise stimulates the machinery in our cells that recycles proteins. This directly targets impaired proteostasis, the hallmark of aging characterized by the accumulation of damaged proteins. Undamaged proteins repair our DNA, which is very important because our DNA is being damaged all the time, and if it's not repaired, it can cause cancer.

Exercise is very good at stimulating autophagy, the process that disassembles damaged proteins and uses the individual elements to make healthy proteins.

THRIVING IN THE
SHADOW OF STRESS

My uncle Ervin Adam seems to be living proof that what doesn't kill us can make us stronger. In his case, strong enough to not just survive tragedies and natural disasters but to lose everything and start over four times and yet be thriving at ninety-seven years and counting. A Czech native, he spent fourteen months in six concentration camps during the Holocaust, and today, he's a self-described "youngster" who still attends lectures two or three times a week at Baylor College of Medicine, where he taught for forty-seven years until retiring at age ninety-four. "I have to keep up," he says in his thick Czech accent, shrugging.

He isn't reluctant to talk about his time in the camps, but he doesn't dwell on the hardship he endured. In fact, when he talks about it, there's the hint of a devilish grin on his face. "When people ask me what I did during World War II, I tell them I made a sightseeing tour of Germany at government expense."

When you ask him why he was moved

around to six camps, he shrugs again. "Because I am a nice fellow. They wanted to show to me more of Germany."

Actually, his reasons for not re-creating his experience are practical. "You couldn't understand. You have no idea. What happened there was unbelievable. It took me twenty-four hours to realize where I was. I didn't know anything about a camp. We never heard about it. But there I was in the middle of it. Fifty years later, how can I explain it so that my grandchildren will believe it? If I was unable to understand it immediately, how can you understand it?"

Even in his autobiography, *Everything Is Otherwise* (Prague, Czechoslovakia Academia, 2018), he devotes only twenty-five pages to his time in the camps and the genocide that he and his sister, Edith, escaped but that claimed his parents' lives. Because he survived and eventually found a peaceful life with his family in the United States, he says, "Auschwitz can be forgotten."

After he was liberated in 1945, he went back to Czechoslovakia and began his medical studies in Prague, with most of his focus on epidemiology and at least a little of his focus on Vlasta Pánková —

soon to be his wife. They both became assistant professors of infectious diseases at Prague's Charles University, but by 1960, they had been kicked off the faculty because they were not Communists. Membership in the Communist Party was a faculty requirement, so Ervin and Vlasta were officially dismissed for providing "insufficient medical-political education" for the university's students.

They had developed expertise regarding polio, though, which led Ervin to a position at Prague's Institute of Immunology and Vlasta to a position at a school for the continuing education of physicians. After the Salk polio vaccine became approved for use in Czechoslovakia in 1958, Uncle Ervin played a critical role in its widespread distribution. The government did not receive enough to vaccinate everyone, so they decided to give it to two-year-old children and hope that they would receive more for the rest of the population. To make the supply go further, Ervin suggested that instead of the standard practice of injecting it into the muscle, one-fifth doses could be injected intradermally (into the second layer of skin) for a sufficient immune response. In

1959, the Czech health service agreed to study the safety and efficacy of this trial with the U.S.-made live polio vaccine, and Ervin was a member of the commission in charge of planning and evaluating the trial. As it turned out, it was so safe and effective that in 1961, Czechoslovakia became the first country to eradicate polio, and for his role, Uncle Ervin received the Award Česká Hlava — the Czech equivalent of a Nobel Prize — in 2012. He and Vlasta also received Gold Medals from Charles University in 1989 for lifetime achievements, and in 2004, Uncle Ervin was elected a foreign member of the Learned Society of the Czech Republic (formerly known as Royal Scientific Society).

And then there was his "second life." In 1968, as the Soviet Army was invading to suppress the liberal reforms of the Prague Spring, he and Vlasta fled with their daughters to Canada, where they stayed a short time before fleeing from violence again. He'd accepted a position at McGill University at a time when Québec separatists were perpetrating bombings in the Montreal area, and when the university became the target of a violent demonstration, he secured a visa and moved the family to Houston, where he joined the faculty at Baylor College of Medicine.

"I'm essentially an adventurer," he says. "It worked out for us, but I would not advise people to do it. If you have a reasonable life standard, if you are not in danger that you are going to lose it, and if you are not a dreamer, sit on your behind where you are. Don't move. It's not easy."

After so many years of adventure, you might think he would have been ready to retire long ago — if not by age sixty-five, at least by seventy-five. But even at eighty-five, "I didn't have the guts to retire," as he puts it. "What would I do in retirement?"

Now that he finally has given up the working life, what does he do to take advantage of the "extra years" he's enjoying?

Like he said, he keeps up. And not just with medicine. He spends two to three hours a day switching back and forth between right-leaning Fox News and left-leaning CNN because "I want to know what is going on in the United States." He also reads Czech weeklies that provide intelligent coverage of

European news and, often, better coverage of U.S. news than he finds in American publications. "They have much better and more authentic comments."

Uncle Ervin is a remarkable example of resilience. Like many SuperAgers, he has suffered the stress of hardship and upheaval and hasn't necessarily abstained from unhealthy habits (he smoked a pipe for twenty-five years). But as surprising as it might seem that Holocaust survivors can thrive for decade after decade and achieve exceptional longevity despite the stress they've endured, in some cases it may be the stress that's responsible, thanks to hormesis. In Uncle Ervin's case, his time in the camps and the flight situations that have been a theme of his life may have upregulated his defense mechanisms to the degree that they've protected him throughout his life.

Hormesis, genes, willpower, or all three? There's also the possibility that a methylation pattern he developed during the Holocaust has protected him ever since. Whatever the answer is, Uncle Ervin is a powerful inspiration for the Einstein team as we uncover the secrets of aging later.

PREVENTING THE LOSS OF MUSCLE MASS AS WE AGE

Exercise is an important component of health throughout our lives but becomes even more important as we age because we become more susceptible to losing muscle and function. Muscle strength, physical performance, and walking speed are commonly used to measure function. Severe muscle loss, called *sarcopenia,* is one of the age-related changes we sometimes see in very old adults because muscle mass is relatively maintained into our forties and then progressively decline. When we look at the biology of aging, we see that the loss of muscle mass occurs because, as we get older, we stop generating enough new muscle cells to compensate for those we have lost. While muscle mass loss is a concern, losing strength is a more significant problem. A decrease in strength can be related to the quality of muscle itself, or it can be caused by vascular and neural changes that occur when an older nervous system doesn't tell the muscles to activate or when oxygen and nutrients are impaired. But this isn't a simple matter to assess, because as people age, they often exercise less and are not as physically active in general, and we know that sedentary behavior can contribute to loss of strength and muscle mass with advancing age.

If left unchecked, muscle loss can lead to poor physical performance, including difficulty with climbing stairs, walking, and rising from a chair, all of which lead to increased risk of falling, disability, and a potential need for long-term medical care. Loss of muscle is also bad for our metabolic health. We start losing muscle mass at about the same age that we see an increase in type 2 diabetes. Muscle is our most important organ for maintaining our sensitivity to insulin, because muscle stores most of the body's sugar as glycogen, and insulin resistance is a primary element of type 2 diabetes. In addition, people usually don't change their eating habits as they age, and when they become less active, they tend to accumulate fat instead of burning those calories.

EXERCISE PLUS METFORMIN

One of the fascinating things we've learned about metformin is that it both activates AMP kinase, which is good for longevity, and inhibits mTOR, which is bad for longevity. To gain greater understanding of what appeared to be a win-win interaction, my friend and collaborator Charlotte Peterson, a gerontologist at the University of Kentucky, conducted an NIH-funded study in which two groups of elderly people did the same amount of strength training for fourteen weeks. During that time, one group took metformin and the other group took a placebo. Charlotte's hypothesis was that since exercise and metformin both activate AMP kinase, together they could be synergistic and amplify the effect. To her surprise, while both groups increased their strength and muscle quality in a clinically significant way, the metformin seemed to inhibit some of the benefits of exercise, in particular the addition of muscle mass. Like in our MILES trial, we studied the tran-scripts — the message that RNA expressed in muscle biopsies obtained before and after exercise in both groups — and we noticed that exercise without metformin and exer-cise with metformin had some similar ef-fects on strength. How can it be that they have less muscle but equal strength? How can it be that, per unit of muscle weight, those who exercised and took metformin performed better than those who only exercised? Ameya Kulkarni, my brilliant former graduate student, noticed that one difference was that members of the met-formin group had less oxidative damage and

290

less inflammation — some of the bad effects of exercise. Also, metformin inhibits mTOR while exercise increases mTOR; the decrease in mTOR may have caused the muscle to function better. At the end of the day, because the subjects did not have different muscle function, the contradictory advantages of exercise and metformin canceled each other out. Although it looked like metformin did not allow all the positive effects of exercise to occur, there's a lot of suggestion that the combination of exercise and metformin has a positive overall effect. In light of this, I take metformin in addition to exercising.

FEEDING OUR LONGEVITY

One in four older Americans is not getting adequate nutrition, and one in three people aged sixty-five and older has diet-related deficiencies. Malnutrition can contribute to decreased strength, weakened immune response, weight loss, anemia, fatigue, mental fog, and confusion. It can also depress thyroid function and increase the risk of harmful drug interactions. So it should be no surprise that older adults who are malnourished see doctors more often and make more trips to the emergency room. They are also hospitalized more often than their peers who are well nourished, and their hospital stays are almost twice as long and cost $2,000–$10,000 more.

Since you're interested in healthy longevity, you probably already know about the ketogenic diet, the Mediterranean diet, and what people who live in blue zones eat. But what may be equally important or even more important for long, healthy lives is what these people do not eat. There's more to good nutrition than following the latest trend, and as with exercise and fasting, dietary recommendations can vary widely depending on individual needs, circumstances, and biological age. But in general, there are five guiding principles to keep in mind:

1. Be Mindful of Your Caloric Intake

Calories matter, so paying attention to how much you eat and choosing to eat just a little less at each meal can make a big difference. We've known for decades that eating less is healthier than eating more.

In a study published by *The Journal of the American Medical Association* that compared decreasing food intake with fasting every other day, the participants in each group lost the same amount of weight on average, but those who fasted said they found it easier than they had found restricting calories on previous diets.

---

1 gram of carbohydrate is about three calories
1 gram of protein is about four calories
1 gram of fat is about nine calories

A gram of fat is the hardest to get rid of, mainly because it has the most calories.

---

2. Get Your Macronutrients

Our bodies use macronutrients, which are the nutrients we get from proteins, fats, carbohydrates, and water, primarily to generate energy and for tissue growth and repair. There's a lot of discussion about the best ratio of proteins, fats, and carbs, but since aging changes biology, that balance is different at different stages of life. For example, we need protein when we're younger, but since it activates mTOR, we've learned that increasing protein for people after a certain biological age is not the right thing to do. But increasing carbohydrates and fat in the aging population isn't ideal either, so there's always some sort of trade-off. The other challenge is that between the ages of sixty and eighty, people in developed countries tend to go from getting too much nutrition to not getting enough. So I don't know that anyone can definitively declare that a particular ratio of macronutrients is optimal at all stages of life.

A questionnaire-based study published in *The Lancet* in 2018 looked at how the ratio of proteins, fats, and carbohydrates affected mortality in 15,428 adults from ages forty-five to sixty-four. The lowest risk of death was for people whose diets were 50–55 percent carbohydrates. For people whose diets were 80 percent carbohydrates, the risk increased by up to 10 percent. And for the people for whom carbs made up 20 percent of their diet, the risk increased by up to 60 percent. So a moderate amount of carbohydrates appears to be better for longevity than a diet that's either high or low in carbs.

But one of the problems with this study is the same problem we have with all diet studies, and that is that people aren't very good at accurately recording what they eat. So whether or not the people with the best results were actually eating 50 percent carbs, we really don't know. Even if they were, we don't know if the results can be attributed to other habits that we are unaware of or cannot measure. As in many studies, the results were statistically adjusted for sex, age, race, total calorie consumption, physical activity, cigarette smoking, diabetes, education, and income level, which all influence mortality. But what if the people with the highest carbohydrate intake were snacking all day long and didn't have enough of a fasting period to regulate the defense against aging? Whatever the case, though, it's safe to assume that a diet that's 65 percent carbohydrates or more is not beneficial.

There is also evidence that people who eat more grain have less mortality than people who eat less grain. But when we take a closer look, we see that they not only were eating more grain but were also eating less beef and might have been getting more exercise than their peers. So the beneficial effects they are experiencing could be from the grains, the exercise, the lower amount of meat, some combination of these factors, or factors we are not even aware of.

Studies also indicate that a diet high in fiber is more important for longevity than a diet low in carbohydrates. High amounts of fiber lower cholesterol, modulate sugar levels, and increase bowel health by keeping things moving through the intestines.

As for protein, studies show that of all the options, meat is the most detrimental to health. In a Loma Linda Adventist Health Study that followed ninety thousand people, those who ate the most meat had about twice as much cardiovascular mortality, while those who ate the most nuts and seeds as their protein sources had 50 percent less mortality. And those who ate less meat and more vegetables had lower body mass indexes, lower incidence of type 2 diabetes, less hypertension, less incidence of cancer, and lower overall mortality.

Processed red meat increased the risk of mortality more than any other protein, but the risk from eating poultry and fish was not significant, and neither was the risk from eating protein from dairy. Eggs appear to increase the mortality rate, though, and there are associations between eating eggs and incidence of cardiovascular mortality. The maximum daily amount of cholesterol recommended in current U.S. guidelines is 200 mg — about the amount contained in one egg. If you increase that to 1,000 mg, you increase your chance of cardiovascular mortality by more than 70 percent, according to a 2019 study reported in *The Journal of the American Medical Association.* Based on the study's results, if you eat two and half eggs a day, you increase your risk of cardiovascular mortality by 40 percent. But maybe the markers we see are actually associated with eating breakfast. Since we typically eat eggs for breakfast, if you skip breakfast, you probably aren't going to have eggs. What would happen if we skipped breakfast and had eggs for dinner? We really don't know, but skipping breakfast keeps looking better.

When we look at nonvegetarians, semi-vegetarians, pesca-vegetarians, lacto-ovo-vegetarians, and vegans, the BMI goes down progressively from 28.8 for nonvegetarians, which is almost obese, to 23.6 for vegans, which is lean. And the incidence of type 2 diabetes goes down from 8 percent in non-vegetarians to 3 percent in vegans. Yet only about 2 percent of our centenarians are vegetarians, again suggesting that genetic factors are important for health span and longevity and that if we identify those, we can protect against the negative effects of our lifestyles and environments.

HYDRATING WISELY

While it's true that water is a macronutrient in the sense that all our organs need it to function, it's also true that we can drink too much of it. Bottled water is more expensive than gasoline, and we don't even know how pure that water is in some cases. We do know that the disposable plastic bottles are adding to our plastic problem worldwide, but beyond bottled water being bad for the planet, we just don't need as much water as the companies selling it want us to believe. In general, men need about four cups of water a day, and women need about three cups. Of course, how much water we need depends on a number of factors, including whether we're exercising and whether we're living in or visiting places that are very dry, have high temperatures, or are located at higher elevations. When we drink excessive amounts of water, we lose sodium. There was a case of water toxicity in a young man because the sodium concentration in his plasma dropped so low that he became unconscious and died. This only happens if your kidneys are not healthy, but how do you know if they are?

It *is* important for the elderly to avoid dehydration, though, and they're a little more prone to it because their biological sensing of thirst declines with age.

PREVENT OBESITY

Obesity contributes to type 2 diabetes and other conditions that can shorten our lives, but while we want to avoid becoming fat, we don't want to stop eating fat because consuming a little of it is good for us and necessary. If you're as pleased as I am to see the words *good* and *fat* together, you're really going to like the news on the ideal body mass index (BMI). While the stereotypical healthy body is lean, studies that have looked at millions of people, at all ages, around the world have determined that the lowest mortality rates are associated with people who probably have some extra subcutaneous fat, and this applies to men and women of all ages. These studies look at BMI and study what BMI levels are most prevalent for mortality. A measurement of 20–24 is considered healthy, below 20 is underweight, above 25 is overweight and 30 or more is obese. Based on these numbers, we might guess that people who have a BMI in the healthy range would have the lowest mortality. But it's actually the overweight people with BMIs around 27. Not too fat — just a little fluffy like me. People with BMIs in this range might also have a little more visceral fat, but our subcutaneous fat is protecting us, and that's probably happening in conjunction with our genetics. Also, high BMI is a strong marker for diabetes, but we don't know if lower BMIs protect against diabetes or if it's the diet that's offering protection.

WHAT'S YOUR BMI?

You can calculate your BMI at https://www .aarp.org/health/healthy-living/info-2017/ bmi_calculator.html

---

As our weight increases, so does our risk for the following conditions:

- Coronary heart disease
- Type 2 diabetes
- Cancers (endometrial, breast, and colon)
- High blood pressure
- High total cholesterol
- High triglycerides levels
- Liver and gallbladder disease
- Sleep apnea and respiratory problems
- Osteoarthritis
- Gynecological problems (abnormal menstruation, infertility)
- Stroke

Losing weight by following a healthy diet can:

- Lower blood pressure
- Make it easier to manage diabetes
- Reduce the risk of cancer
- Reduce bad (LDL) cholesterol levels

While there are important benefits to losing weight, carrying a few extra pounds after we're age sixty-five may reduce our risk of disability and increase our longevity.

3. Support Our Microscopic "Friends"

We have more microbial cells — about thirty-nine trillion total — than other cells. These bacteria cells make up our microbiomes, and just like our fingerprints, microbiomes are unique for each person. When people hear the word *microbiome,* they tend to think of the good bacteria that live in our guts, but these microbial cells are everywhere in our bodies as well as outside it, on our skin. We have known about these cells for some time, and we have known that the microbiome in the intestine is important for processing vitamins A, D, E, and K, but until recently, we were not aware of the profound effects it can have on all systems of the body or its link to many age-related diseases and depression. Several studies, including the NIH's Human Microbiome Project, have looked at the relationship between our microbiomes and our health spans and life spans, but we still don't know how microbes affect the biology of aging. That's likely to change soon because numerous experiments aimed at curing a variety of illnesses and diseases by altering the gut's microbiome are under way. So far, we have evidence linking the health of the microbiome with digestion, immune response, inflammation, bone density, and cognition.

Although we have more questions than answers, there is no doubt that the microbiome is an important part of our physiology. And when we do experiments in our laboratory by transplanting microbacteria or administering antibiotics in decreasing doses, we can see that there are significant physiological effects. But my biggest interest is in whether the microbiome plays a major role in aging. From what we have seen, the microbiome does not change significantly in aging adults unless they are in hospitals or institutions or they are getting antibiotics, but that doesn't mean that there aren't individual differences between balanced and imbalanced microbiomes.

TRILLIONS OF "MOUTHS" TO FEED

The microbiome in the gut seems to benefit from the live bacteria cultures in yogurt and fermented vegetables such as sauerkraut. It appears not to favor antibiotics, laxatives, artificial sweeteners, processed food, or a sedentary lifestyle.

4. Eat for Optimal Health, Not to Lose Weight

Of all the popular diets that have been in fashion over the years, the only one that was based on a clinical study with interventions and a control group and that has proved to increase health span and life span in humans is the Mediterranean diet. In PREDIMED, a long-term study conducted in Spain, 7,500 men and women who were slightly overweight and at risk for diabetes and heart disease were randomly divided into two groups and studied for five years. One group ate the low-fat diet that was being recommended in the West when the study began, and the other group ate a high-fat Mediterranean diet that was supplemented with either almonds or olive oil. Although many doctors said that olive oil was extremely unhealthy because it was high in calories and a mix of saturated and unsaturated fats, the people in the study who consumed the olive oil had the best results, just slightly better than those who supplemented their diet with almonds. Compared with the group that ate the low-fat diet, those who ate the Mediterranean diet had a third less diabetes, heart disease, and stroke, and they had less cognitive decline. As a bonus, they also lost some weight.

Keep in mind that results like these are rarely attributed to a single factor or a single food. The Mediterranean diet includes a wide variety of vegetables and fruits, whole grains and legumes, small amounts of fish and poultry, and very little red meat. But the olive oil did appear to be the most significant element in the study results. People in Spain, Greece, and Italy, on average, consume more than three gallons of extra-virgin olive oil a year, compared with people in the United States, who average about a quart a year. So people in the Mediterranean are getting twelve times more of this liquid gold than Americans.

ALL OLIVE OIL IS NOT ALIKE

Olive oil's antioxidant polyphenols have a direct effect on blood vessels and genes, and they feed the good gut bacteria and produce fatty acids that lower inflammation.

In the PREDIMED study, only the extra-virgin olive oil delivered health benefits. Olive oils that were not extra-virgin did not appear to produce any benefits. Cold-pressed extra-virgin olive oil contains about thirty types of polyphenols that reduce inflammation and target the hallmarks of aging, particularly in the cardiovascular system and the brain. It also has lower acidity and tastes better than less healthy olive oils.

If you are concerned that olive oil might produce carcinogens when you cook with it, no negative health consequences were observed among the people in the study who regularly cooked with it.

NUTRACEUTICALS ARE IN THE WORKS

We're already seeing some healthier snack options on supermarket shelves, and we'll see more of them in the coming years. Nutraceuticals and truly healthy snacks are some of the newest products in the works at food production companies. When Pepsi asked the members of its scientific advisory board on which I served to help figure out the types of healthy snacks that would meet the needs of the elderly, we were advised to think outside of the box.

"Well," I said, "my first recommendation is that you buy Guinness beer. It has lots of nutrients, and besides that, if you give it to the elderly, they'll be happy, too."

We laughed, knowing that was never going to happen, but it was a good way to begin the explanation of how nutritional needs change as we age. In general, between the ages of sixty and eighty, people go from being overweight or obese to being thin and malnourished (although their abdominal fat seems to stay the same). This happens at different rates for different people, so the recommendations for best snacks change with aging. Many people who are eighty and older and losing weight can benefit from some high-calorie snacks.

Older people are also losing muscle and proteins, but giving them protein can activate the anti-longevity protein mTOR. (Incidentally, the drug rapamycin blocks mTOR and extends life span.) So high-protein snacks that can be good for younger people may not be a good choice for older people, and neither are snacks that are high in sugar or salt. As a result, elderly people's options for healthy packaged snacks are a little limited, but discussion is continuing.

5. Supplement Only as Needed and Without Doing Harm: Micronutrients and Vitamins

We need micronutrients because they play subtle but vital biochemical and physiological roles in cellular processes, including nerve conduction and vascular functions. As we age, our bodies aren't as efficient at absorbing and using vitamins and minerals, so our need for micronutrients increases. Many older adults are taking medication, and some medications can also interfere with the absorption of nutrients. These factors combined mean that having a nutrition-rich diet becomes even more important as we age. While younger, healthy people can get their nutrient requirements entirely from food and rarely need supplements, this is often not the case for older people, especially if they're sick. But some vitamins taken in excess or in combination with certain drugs can be harmful. Combining exercise with large amounts of vitamins, such as vitamin E, has even been fatal.

There are some vitamins that, when taken correctly, do not do harm, and for people who have true deficiencies, they may be helpful. For example, when elderly people are losing weight and starting to decline, supplementing their diets with complex vitamins and minerals is considered a safe and beneficial practice. But many people who are age fifty or older may also need to boost their intake of vitamin B12, calcium, and vitamin D.

Check with your doctor to find out if you need more:

Vitamin B12
We need vitamin B12 to keep our nerve cells and red blood cells healthy.

Rich sources: liver and kidneys, especially from lamb, clams, sardines, beef, trout, salmon, and eggs. But older people may not absorb enough of it from food. B12 is also deficient in some patients who have been taking metformin for a long time. I have lower B12 levels and take monthly B12 shots.

Calcium

As people age, bones start to lose calcium at an increased rate, and since calcium is a critical ingredient for bone strength and resistance to fractures, it's very important to get enough.

Rich sources: green leafy vegetables like broccoli, collard greens, kale, and spinach, low-fat dairy products, and nondairy "milk" that's fortified with calcium. But as with vitamin B12, older adults may not absorb enough of this micronutrient from food.

Vitamin D

Vitamin D helps calcium to work, and low levels of vitamin D are associated with a high risk of diseases, so the best thing we can do is expose our skin to more sunlight. Older people aren't always able to get enough vitamin D in this way, so many are deficient in it. And while vitamin D supplements have shown results with the prevention of fractures in women with osteoporosis, we have not seen dramatic results from supplementation in other studies. Some supplements like vitamin D won't hurt us, but too much of some vitamins including vitamin E can be harmful, so supplementation should be done under the direction of your doctor.

Rich sources: Sunlight on skin is the only source that we know works. Vitamin D–fortified low-fat milks may help.

THE MAGIC PILLS
WE'VE BEEN WISHING FOR

When I treat people who are struggling to lose weight, they often say things like, "There should be a pill I can take that lets me eat as much as I want without getting fat." Not too long ago, this idea appeared to be a pipe dream, but not anymore. The race to develop pharmaceuticals and nutraceuticals that mimic the benefits of caloric restriction is already under way. Some drugs will cause weight loss, while others will mimic the advantages of caloric restriction without causing weight loss and will be appropriate for people who are not obese.

With this in mind, researchers are studying the tiny compounds of molecules called *metabolites* that circulate in our blood. These compounds are made of amino acids, sugars, and fats, and we're studying the roles they play in longevity. There are thousands of metabolites of interest, and my colleague Derek Huffman looked at four hundred metabolites that can be measured in plasma. We were looking for metabolites with levels that decrease with age, and we wanted to see if those levels would return to more normal "youthful" levels when we restricted the mice's calories.

With my funding, Derek began the study with four groups of rats, two of which — one made up of young rats and the other made up of old rats — could eat as much as they wanted. Groups three and four were young rats with restricted diets and old rats with restricted diets. In collaboration with Daniel Promislow, a computation biologist at University of Washington, we identified a metabolite called *sarcosine* that appeared to be a longevity superhero. In rats, sarcosine levels declined with age, but when we restricted their diets, they went up in both the young and the old. This is exactly the response we were looking for as we went through each of those hundreds of metabolites. Then we decided to measure sarcosine in humans. First, we collaborated with geriatrician Luigi Fontana, then at Washington University, who follows the CRONies, and we compared the metabolites of young and old CRONies with those of a control group of young and old people. We got exactly the same results as we got in rats; in the control group, sarcosine was high in young people

311

and went down with age. Sarcosine declined slightly with age in the CRONies, but it remained higher than the sarcosine levels in the control group.

Next, we needed to find the cellular mechanism that's implicated by which sarcosine targets aging. At Einstein, when Ana Maria Cuervo, codirector of our institute, administered sarcosine to animals and examined what happened with the cells' ability to carry out autophagy, which becomes less efficient with age, the sarcosine significantly enhanced one of the processes of autophagy in the same way that caloric restriction in animals enhances this process. Ana Maria is a member of the American Academy of Arts and Sciences and the National Academy of Sciences and one of the best scientists and colleagues I could hope for, and together we proceeded to our next experiment.

The next question was how to capitalize on our discovery that sarcosine is something that declines with age but remains higher with caloric restriction. Sarcosine is found in such natural sources as turkey, ham, egg yolks, vegetables, and legumes, but it may be difficult to get enough of it through our diets alone. Since sarcosine is a nutraceutical, however, it could be available immediately, and the results could be astounding. Derek is also looking at drugs that will target the sarcosine pathway and cause an increase in its levels.

WHEN WE EAT MATTERS

In recent years, we have learned that health and longevity are affected not only by what we eat and don't eat but also by when we eat and how long we fast between meals.

There's a lot of ongoing research about fasting, and what we're learning is so promising that I'm experimenting with fasting myself. There are different schools of thought on how we should fast and for how long; at the moment, it's commonly thought that the best results occur when the fast is done for sixteen to twenty-four hours at least once or twice a week, but this recommendation isn't based on much data from humans. To enhance our understanding of the effects of intermittent fasting, Rajat Singh, a molecular pharmacologist at Einstein, is trying to determine the minimum amount of time we need to fast to enhance the biological processes that protect us against aging hallmarks such as impaired autophagy. I'm fasting for sixteen hours a day because that's how long it appears to take for our bodies to use up stored sugar called *glycogen.* Then insulin levels drop to adapt to the presence of less sugar and enhance the liver's ability to provide as much glucose as needed. When there is less insulin, there is less mTOR and more autophagy. While insulin levels are low, the body taps into its fat storage, and fat is released into the bloodstream. When those fats reach the liver, they are turned into energy molecules called *ketones,* which appear to sustain us through the stress. And while there isn't much scientific data on how a ketone-rich diet affects humans, it has been shown to extend life span in animals. We are also looking at how ketones affect cardiovascular health, blood pressure, LDL cholesterol, triglycerides, and insulin sensitivity, so ketones may play a big role as we study the benefits of fasting for humans.

Although it's not practical for everyone, based on what we learned from our caloric restriction experiments at Einstein, fasting daily may generally produce the best results. Initially, we thought that restricting calories was responsible for the positive results we were seeing — the animals' health span was improved, and their mid and maximal life span increased significantly. But since we had been feeding them only once a day, we realized that the results were more about fasting than restricting calories! And in recent studies, the calorically restricted rats that were fed a limited number of calories throughout the day were lean like the calorically restricted rats that ate all their food in the morning. But the rats that ate throughout the day did not live as long, and the rats that ate once a day also demonstrated better cognition and retained their physical functions for much longer than the other rats. So based on such studies, it looks like how often we eat and how long we fast are more important than restricting calories. And for many people, including myself, it's also easier to do than counting calories.

Thanks to research that AFAR has supported, new findings about the advantages of fasting in animal studies have led to a variety of fasting programs that are being tested with people to see if the effects are as profound as they are in animals. Biogerontologist Valter Longo suggests doing a five-day fasting-mimicking diet three or four times a year. In his book *The Longevity Diet,* Valter explains that the foods we eat affect us at a cellular level. Our cells all have nutrient sensors that can switch hundreds of genes on or off, depending on what we eat. Some nutrients are more triggering for those sensors than others are, so Valter created diets with foods that avoid triggering them. In this way, the diet mimics fasting, and with mice, these diets have been successful in reversing diabetes. Another lifestyle guru, my friend Peter Attia, M.D., does zero fasting, a seven-day fast with almost no calories, four times a year.

Other fasting-related research is focused on the times that we eat and how they are in line with our bodies' natural rhythms — or not. Circadian rhythms are the day-to-night, light-to-dark cycles that affect all people and animals. Satchin Panda, an expert on circadian rhythm research at the Salk Institute, has found that aligning our eating with these rhythms is one pathway to good health. In *The Circadian Code,* he explains that having our meals between early morning and early evening is healthier than eating all day long and then snacking at night. Essentially, you would fast for fourteen to sixteen hours under this plan, so it shares a number of commonalities with intermittent fasting. With mice, restricting calorie intake to eight to ten hours a day has improved their health even when they were eating a diet high in fat and sugar. In humans, short-term studies have shown that intermittent fasting is an effective way to control weight, and it seems to have many benefits beyond weight loss.

All these programs have merit, but fasting for at least sixteen hours is showing the most promise for life span and health span, which is why I'm doing it. I have also lost some weight, but that's just a nice side effect, not the reason I started this practice. When I share my personal example with people, it surprises me that so many of them think I'm harming myself by skipping breakfast. "Breakfast is the most important meal of the day!" they assure me. But guess what — there is no scientific evidence to support that, and in fact, if you're trying to lose weight, skipping breakfast might be a good idea. Several valid studies have concluded that eating breakfast can lead to weight gain. When you think about it, it's not likely that breakfast was part of the plan for our prehistoric ancestors, who spent the day hunting, fishing, and gathering grains, seeds, nuts, and small fruits. It's not as if Wheaties or Special K were available in the morning, and it's safe to say that nobody was obese. The carb-heavy morning meal did not become popular until modern times. Bottom line: Infants and children may benefit by eating breakfast, but for adults, it's not biologically necessary, and skipping it as part of intermittent fasting may contribute to a longer, healthier life.

What About Sleep?

Sleep is often grouped with diet and exercise as one of the three keys to good health, so we expected to see a link between sufficient sleep and longevity, but our research did not show that link. Some of our centenarians report sleeping an average of eight hours a night and napping during the day — a nice amount of sleep — and we thought that might be a factor in their longevity, but it turned out that some of them are napping because they don't sleep well at night. Lavy Klein, a visiting professor from Israel, analyzed our sleep data and did find something else that was interesting, though — the centenarians in our study appear to have longevity genes that protect them from diseases associated with sleep disorders, so whether they're sleeping enough or not, they are not getting those diseases.

Among the centenarians' offspring and the control group, a significant number of people regularly experience sleep disturbances, and many in the control group have diabetes, cardiovascular disease, and other diseases linked to sleep deprivation while the centenarians' offspring do not. So while longevity genes are not insurance against sleep disturbances themselves, they do appear to protect against their worst effects. For those of us who were not born with the longevity genes, though, it certainly makes sense to sleep as well as we can to head off the diseases that can result from sleep disorders and deprivation.

In 2017, the Nobel Prize in Physiology or Medicine was awarded to Jeffrey C. Hall, Michael Rosbash, and Michael W. Young for figuring out how biological clocks work by doing research with fruit flies. Biological clocks keep flies, fish, frogs, plants, and people on schedules that are about twenty-four hours long whether we know if it's day or night or not. Our biological clocks are run by "clock genes" that make a protein when they're turned on. Once a particular amount of the protein accumulates, it turns the clock genes off. But the protein degrades with time, and when it drops to a certain level, the clock genes switch back on. The cycle affects nearly all our bodies' systems.

The scientists were initially surprised to discover that the clock genes don't just exist in the brain — they found them in many parts of the fly. And now we know that we have these clock genes throughout our bodies. In addition to our brains, our hearts, lungs, livers, and other organs have the genes. They even exist within individual cells, and that's why cells tend to do repair work and cell division at certain times. These findings have very promising implications. For example, they suggest it might be more effective to take medications or treatments at certain times rather than others.

We are also seeing that animals with the best clock genes may live longer. In one study, the mice that had the most reliable clock genes — the ones that maintained a twenty-four-hour-day cycle even in total darkness — outlived the mice that had clocks that did not maintain such a regular cycle.

We have known for some time that people whose sleep patterns are disrupted by working night shifts are at higher risk for a variety of conditions and diseases than people who work during the day and sleep at night. Over time, night shift workers tend to experience more ulcers, heart disease, diabetes, and cancer. They also experience more insomnia, depression, and dementia. And Ana Maria Cuervo's research has shown that the clock genes change autophagy, like a garbage disposal, and that activating autophagy activates clock genes. Once we learn more about clock genes and how they work, we will be able to time medical treatments and interventions so they have the most positive benefits. Meanwhile, drug developers are exploring medications that might offer protection against sleep disturbances and irregular schedules.

OUR DNA HAS SOMETHING TO SAY

Another way we can increase our chances for longer health spans and life spans is by taking steps to offset genetic mechanisms with lifestyle choices and — when they become available — new drugs that will be designed to specifically target those mechanisms. What we need to keep in mind is that genetic information is in no way a diagnosis, and many times, it is not even a strong indicator that we may develop particular diseases or conditions later in life. But it can offer some helpful information, and that's why so many companies are offering genetic testing. For example, 23andMe provides ancestry information and also gives you the option to learn about your DNA with regard to health and longevity. Not everyone wants to know about their genes, and we have to respect that, but for those who do want to know, these types of tests may help us to delay or stop the potential onset of diseases. If a woman has the BRCA1 mutation that's associated with a very high risk for breast cancer, for instance, and her mother, sisters, and aunts have had cancer, she may decide to eliminate her risk by having her breasts and ovaries removed relatively early in life. And people with the APOE4 genotype, which is a strong predictor of Alzheimer's, may qualify to participate in studies testing drugs that can prevent cognitive decline.

But while these two genotypes are associated with diseases in many studies, we still have to look at their predictive values. In other words, if you have a particular genotype, what are your chances of getting the associated disease? The answer to that question isn't clear. While BRCA1 has a very high penetrance — the proportion of people with a gene variant associated with breast cancer — most genotypes have undetermined penetrance. So at least for now, genetic tests are not as good at predicting diseases as lab tests that measure cholesterol, glucose, and blood pressure.

Remember that when we did gene sequencing with forty-four of our first centenarians, they had more than 230 genotypes that were associated with diseases they did not have because they also have other differences that protect them from the hallmarks of aging. We have also seen the CETP genotype associated with both improved cognitive function and cognitive decline, and we've seen that CETP's effects are not universal. So part of the challenge is that it's never about a single genotype. In fact, looking at genotypes in isolation makes no sense because we're not built from one variant at a time, but that's how we analyze the information. We're built from many, many variants, and some of them can cancel each other out, and some of them can amplify each other. It's so complex that genetic testing is not always predictive, but it can give us a chance to be proactive. If you do choose to have genetic testing done, be sure the results are being interpreted in ways that put the finding into context, because getting genetic information without a clear explanation or without counseling can be unnecessarily stressful.

In the case of my own genetic testing, I found out that I'm at "risk" for having perfect pitch. My son and daughter, who both play the piano, have tested me and say it seems to be true. It's possible that if my parents had known that when I was young, they would have encouraged me to pursue a career in music, and I may not be a doctor writing a book today but a conductor.

While that information was mostly just entertaining, I did learn something else that might provide a clue to why I tend to test low for vitamin D. The test said I had a slight risk for lactose intolerance. I don't suffer when I eat cheese, and I love it, so I still eat it, but it's possible that eating dairy may speed up my digestive system's transit time, and that could mean my body doesn't have enough time to absorb the vitamin D. Whatever the case, I take vitamin D supplements because they might help and won't hurt.

A concern I hear about DNA testing is that the results might prevent people from getting insurance coverage if the preexisting conditions clause is eliminated or could work against them in some other way. Keep in mind that this information is private, and while it can be predictive, there are way too many variables to conclude that any genetic variant in and of itself is going to result in the associated disease. Even in the case of the BRCA1 gene with its high penetrance, not everyone is going to get cancer. Your cholesterol and glucose levels, blood pressure, and family history for diseases are much more predictive than genotype, and your doctor and insurance company already have that information, so disclosing a genotype is usually not going to put you at additional risk.

PREVENTION MATTERS

The following diagnostic tests and vac-
cines are recommended:

DIAGNOSTIC TESTS

We know that biological age and chronological age differ, but to be on the safe
side, we should have all these tests by
the time we're fifty.

Blood Glucose/HbA1C
Blood Pressure
Colonoscopy
HDL and LDL Cholesterol and
  Triglycerides
Mammogram
Pap Smear
Prostate Cancer Check

VACCINES

Flu Shots*
Pneumococcal
Shingles
Td/Tdap

*Although we encourage the elderly to get
flu shots, they often don't, because many
of them know that it doesn't guarantee

that they won't get the flu. Most immunization protects people completely, but the immunization for the flu is about 40 percent effective and possibly only 20 percent effective in the elderly population. But I still recommend flu shots for the elderly, because if they get the flu, many of them will need to be hospitalized, and they dislike that more than most things.

STAY MENTALLY SHARP

Aerobic exercise and diet may have as much of an effect — and possibly even more of an effect — on keeping our minds clear and sharp as brain workouts do. Everyone knows that exercise is good for the body, but we didn't know how good it was for the brain. Recent studies suggest that exercise may be even more important than staying mentally engaged when it comes to staving off cognitive decline and dementia. And we're also learning more about the link between nutrition and cognition.

Epidemiologist and clinical dietitian Claire McEvoy is working toward increasing our understanding of how diet affects cognitive health as we age. She's looking specifically at the Mediterranean diet and other heart-healthy dietary habits because what's good for the heart often proves to be good for the brain, too. When she looked at the Mediterranean diet as part of the Health and Retirement Study and the Coronary Artery Risk Development in Young Adults study, she found that both older and younger people who ate this way had better cognitive health. Another study found that eating the Mediterranean diet as young adults can help to keep cognitive function stronger at midlife.

Based on these and other similar studies, what we eat may have cumulative protective effects on our brain function throughout our lives. If so, eating well throughout our lives can help to slow the onset of cognitive decline and may reduce the risk of dementia later in life. High-quality diets such as the Mediterranean diet also have anti-inflammatory and antioxidant effects, and these effects may also help to protect from dementia and Alzheimer's as we age. But this quest is far from over. We still have a lot to discover and learn before we'll be able to recommend an optimal combination of nutrients and foods for lifelong brain health.

Researchers are also looking for connections between sleep and brain health. While the connections between mental health and sleep aren't as clear as those between mental health and exercise and nutrition, we're starting to gain more understanding in this area. Researchers, including Kristine Yaffe, a neuropsychiatrist from the University of California–San Francisco School of Medicine, has been looking at how disrupted sleep might contribute to dementia. A study published in the journal *Sleep* found that people whose sleep was often disrupted had a 1.68 times greater risk for cognitive impairment, including Alzheimer's, than people who slept well. But the researchers were careful to point out that it's not clear whether sleep disorders cause cognitive decline or are a symptom of it. A study published in *Science* in 2019 connects more of the dots, though. Researchers David M. Holtzman, M.D., and Brendan P. Lucey, M.D., explored how a lack of sleep is connected to an increase in two proteins associated with Alzheimer's. One of the proteins, called *tau,* was also found in excess in adults who were extremely sleep-deprived. Other reports on sleep-deprived adults showed that the protein amyloid-beta (A-beta) was present in their brains in high levels, and this protein is also seen in excess in the brains of people who have Alzheimer's disease.

In one study, eight adults were monitored during a night of normal sleep and also over the span of thirty-six hours without sleep. Samples of their cerebrospinal fluid showed a 51.5 percent increase in the tau protein (a biomarker for Alzheimer's disease) in participants who were deprived of sleep. This was similar to the results of a study done with mice in which the sleep-deprived mice had twice as much tau as the mice that slept. Since both tau and A-beta increase when we don't get enough sleep, researchers are looking at how treating sleep disorders in midlife and finding treatments to help people get enough sleep can decrease the risk for Alzheimer's. While we sleep, the brain seems to dispose of debris, including excess proteins, so it's possible that when we don't get adequate sleep, our disposal systems don't have enough time to do their jobs.

While the connections between sleep and staying mentally sharp are still being researched, we do know that there is a clear association in older adults between getting good sleep and psychological well-being. But we haven't seen the same connection between quantity of sleep and psychological well-being. So if you're sleeping less as you age but still feeling good during the day, sleeping less may be normal for you. But if you're sleeping poorly and it's affecting what you can do during the day or making you feel impatient or anxious, you should discuss the changes with your doctor.

Mental Engagement
Can Preserve Cognition

The Advanced Cognitive Training for Independent and Vital Elderly (ACTIVE) study led by George W. Rebok of the Johns Hopkins Center on Aging and Health, suggests that reasoning, memory, and how fast thoughts can be processed can be maintained with cognitive training. In this study with 2,832 participants, those who engaged in mental exercises maintained these abilities for ten years longer than the control group. Our SuperAgers attend lectures, work crossword puzzles, use modern technology, and actively engage with the world around them. Drugs are being tested that will give us all the same genetic edge that they have, but in the meantime, it's a good idea to keep your brain "in shape." My colleague Joe Verghese, Einstein's chief of geriatrics and a partner in some of our grants, has shown that mental engagement such as working crossword puzzles delays cognitive decline. New types of brain exercises and games that can help to preserve memory and the speed that our brains process thoughts are in the works, although so far there's little evidence that supports some of the claims being made by the producers and manufacturers. But there is sophisticated technology that combines virtual reality with brain imaging that can show where and how various types of training can activate the brain and lead to improved memory.

In other promising research, Adam Gazzaley, M.D., Ph.D., and director of the Neuroscience Imaging Center at the University of California–San Francisco, and his team observed that when adults aged sixty to eighty-five were trained on a game called Neuroracer, they experienced improvements in their abilities to multitask, their working memories, and their abilities to sustain attention that lasted for six months or more. This study shows that some computer games may be more effective than some of the traditional brain-training games done with pencil and paper, but before buying these new products, be sure to investigate the claims to see if quality research backs them up.

At Einstein, we use a variety of tests to measure cognition; Joe designed one that you can do at home called Walking While Talking. In it, he asks elderly people to walk twenty or thirty feet at their regular pace. Then he asks them to talk while they walk and observes whether they slow down. They're walking slowly to begin with, so when they slow down, it's not because they're getting winded or tired — it's because our ability to multitask declines with age. The next test is to ask them to solve simple math problems as they walk, and those tests become progressively more mentally challenging. In this way, we can find out which tasks are slowing them down the most and what parts of cognition they need the most support with.

Keep in mind that doing poorly on some of these tests does not mean that someone has dementia. It just means they have abilities they need to compensate for or approach differently, and multitasking is usually one of them. But it's important to keep in mind that while some abilities of older adults decline, other abilities emerge. Dr. Tsvi Lanir in Israel found that older people's brains become biologically wiser. They can see the end point faster and take shortcuts to get there, so in this way their mental processing is faster than younger people's. Older people's brains also have gained the ability to modulate their emotional responses, which is why they tend not to overreact and often become peace seekers.

Harness the Power of Purpose

There is a significant amount of data from scientific studies that suggests that people who have a strong sense of purpose are healthier and enjoy a higher quality of life than people who do not. In one study, researchers wanted to find out if there is a link between having a life purpose and mortality among older people in the United States.

Based on data from 6,985 adults from ages fifty to sixty-one and their spouses of varying ages, the Health and Retirement Study found that people with a strong purpose in life lived longer than people who did not. The researchers also concluded that living purposefully may have health benefits. Since life purpose is a mortality risk factor that people can change, future research will be looking for methods and practices that can help people to identify and strengthen their life purposes. It will also be interesting to see if life purpose affects health through biological mechanisms. As long as you have more plans than achievements, you'll probably be hanging in here for a while.

Focus on the Positive

Positive attitude was the fourth most common reason the SuperAgers thought they lived longer than their peers, and we were curious to see if the science would support that theory. So we decided to look at whether a positive attitude toward life, together with some other psychological factors like emotional expression, could be a factor in exceptional longevity. For this study, Kaori Kato, a student at the Ferkauf Graduate School of Psychology at the time, developed a brief personality measure to characterize the centenarians. The results showed that the group of centenarians had a positive attitude toward life — they were optimistic, easygoing, outgoing, and laughed often. They expressed emotions instead of bottling them up and had significantly less depression and anxiety than the control group. They also scored higher than the control group in extroversion, agreeability, and conscientiousness. Kato's findings suggested that the presence of certain personality characteristics may be associated with favorable cognitive and mental health outcomes in advanced age, but the findings do not show whether the centenarians had had a positive attitude throughout life or if it developed later in life. So we don't know if this great personality that we saw at one hundred had anything to do with their reaching that age.

This became obvious one day after I met with a new centenarian in our study. Max was 104, extroverted, optimistic, and very agreeable, and he had nothing but kind things to say about all his family members. I had fun talking with him and thoroughly enjoyed our time together. Shortly after our visit, I bumped into his son, who is also in our study, and told him his father was one of the nicest guys I'd ever met. The son laughed. "You should have seen the son of a bitch when he was my age," he said. "He was terrible."

That's when I wondered how many of the delightful centenarians had been less pleasant when they were younger. What had happened to the one I'd just met to change him from "terrible" at age eighty to terrific twenty years later? We really don't know much about the aging brain beyond the age of eighty, but there have been studies that suggest that older people pay more attention to the positive than the negative and remember more of the positive, too. In a study comparing the recollection ability of young people and older people, University of Pennsylvania researchers showed the subjects a wide range of slide images, from very pleasing images like a beach at sunset to disturbing images like a pizza crawling with cockroaches. The young people recalled it all — the good, the bad, and the ugly. But the older people mainly recalled the pleasing slides, which suggests there's some biology at work when it comes to our enjoyment of the aging process.

There is ongoing research regarding mind-set and health, and in 2019, *JAMA* published a study that found that being optimistic was associated with a lower risk of cardiovascular events, while being pessimistic was linked to a higher risk of these events. These findings came by way of a meta-analysis of fifteen studies that included 229,391 participants. This information is very promising, because mind-set is something that can potentially be changed and may become a new focus for clinical intervention.

OTHER PROMISING PRACTICES

There are many practices that appear to be beneficial and have been safely employed for many years. Practices like yoga, meditation, guided visualization, and reflexology are doing good things for people, and some people swear by the healing powers of listening to certain types of music, singing, or chanting. Others say that creating artwork or expressing themselves through dance keeps them feeling inspired or has helped them to heal. Just because we don't know how the biology of something works doesn't mean it's not beneficial, so practices that can enhance health and happiness without the risk of doing harm are worth exploring.

What I Do

In just about every interview I do, I'm asked what I do myself to stay young. I'm happy to share that with you, but only with the caveat that what works for me may not be the right things for you.

Exercise

I started exercising regularly mainly so I could eat more of the great food I love. But later, I learned that exercising does not have as much impact on weight loss as eating less. If you exercise for thirty minutes, you can burn about three hundred calories. But if you reduce your daily food intake by 20 percent, you eliminate about six hundred calories. But exercise helps us to stay younger at any age and no matter what our condition, so I've made it part of my everyday life.

Aerobic:

Almost every day, I run three miles on my treadmill or I bike ten miles. I also take advantage of the new technology and track my steps with a Fitbit and an iPhone. I think it's motivating to keep track and even though we don't know that ten thousand steps a day is the minimum requirement, I'd rather do more than the minimum.

Strength Training:
Once a week

Balance and Flexibility:
Once a week with a trainer

Nutrition

I try not to overdo it with carbs or dessert, but for the most part, I eat anything I want for dinner and put off eating the next day for as long as I can. That may mean having a late lunch or not eating until dinner, but I make sure I stay hydrated with water and noncaloric drinks, including tea and coffee. If I need a snack, I eat several almonds or olives but very few carbohydrates that are poorly absorbed. I often fast on consecutive days, eating only in the evening, and I've been surprised by how easy it is and how well I feel.

I have also been monitoring my glucose levels with FreeStyle Libre 14 day system. It's a tiny patch that holds a needle that's implanted in the back of my arm and a monitor about half the size of an iPhone. I don't see or feel the needle, and it doesn't affect anything I do. When I want to know what my blood sugar is, all I have to do is turn on the monitor and hold it over my arm. I was curious to see what happened with my glucose levels after fasting and exercising and how the levels changed based on what I ate, and some of the readings have surprised me. For example, after fasting for seventeen hours, I ate a tuna salad sandwich on rye bread, and my glucose levels shot up to 170, which is quite high. If I'd had a blood test at that moment, the results would have said I was diabetic. After this experience, I was worried about what my glucose level would be after I ate my favorite meal — chicken paprikash. To my pleasant surprise, the meal barely budged my glucose level after I'd fasted for sixteen hours! So this is just another example of how personal nutrition is and why we need to monitor how we feel after eating or not eating certain foods.

Supplements

NMN

I take NMN, which is a precursor of an energy mediator called *NAD+*. (*NMN* stands for *nicotinamide mononucleotide* and is believed to activate genes that are related to longevity.) We can't live without the coenzyme NAD+ (nicotinamide adenine dinucleotide), and studies have indicated that NAD+ appears to decline with age. David Sinclair and others have shown the health benefits of mice that were fed NMN or other NAD+ precursors. They could run longer than the mice that didn't get this supplement, stayed healthier for longer, and died later. As a physician, I didn't want to do anything that had not been proved in a double-blind study, but when I turned sixty-two, I decided I should include some things in my diet that I believe are safe, even if we don't have all the answers yet.

The one thing that I noticed with taking NMN is that, according to my Fitbit, my REM sleep has become better.

Aspirin

I've been taking aspirin for thirty years even though recent studies have not documented its effectiveness in preventing heart attacks, strokes, or even colon cancer. In fact, a big trial showed that aspirin may be harmful in people who are over the age of seventy, but I take it because I fly frequently and want to protect myself from deep vein thrombosis.

Sleep

I try to get seven hours of sleep every night, and my Fitbit also gives me information about my sleeping patterns. This is helpful because sometimes I don't feel like I've slept well, but the Fitbit indicates I have. The sensation of not feeling well rested can occur if we wake up while we're dreaming.

Staying Mentally Sharp

Every day, my life is filled with interesting questions and pursuits, so I'm always thinking.

HOW TO DECIDE
WHAT'S GOOD FOR YOU

The internet teems with the latest news on how to stay young, but many of those stories are incomplete or misleading. Although learning how to cut through the noise and decipher what's real science and what isn't can seem daunting, doing due diligence and discussing new research with your doctor

341

will help you to determine how the news might be beneficial for you. The information I have shared is limited to practices and treatments that have been rigorously tested, and I have also touched on some possibilities that are promising and should not do harm. But again, choices should always be made on an individual basis.

Make sure there's scientific research to back up claims, as well as clinical studies done with humans, and find out who funded the research. If a study is supported by organizations like AFAR and NIH that are dedicated to real science, they have merit. But many studies are tilted toward a particular outcome and therefore don't meet the criteria that reputable journals like *JAMA* require before publishing them.

You also want to explore any associated side effects. Even some of the safest supplements and herbs can become dangerous in combination with certain pharmaceuticals or procedures. If there is any chance that a treatment or a drug can do harm, be sure to discuss it with your doctor.

NINE:
BRIGHT HORIZONS

Space-age technologies, designer drugs that target the hallmarks of aging, and life-changing longevity research are already in the works. Because of these innovations, people will stay healthy for an additional ten to twenty years, and the most common side effect will be living to one hundred and beyond. The time line still needs to be determined, but chances are, children who are in elementary school now will live long enough to meet their great-great-grandchildren. New technologies not only are changing the ways we treat illness and disease but are also providing us with revolutionary options for early detection of diseases and, better yet, early detection of the hallmarks of aging, which precede sickness and disease. New technology, including artificial intelligence, is making it possible for us to study thousands of data points at a time rather than having to take

343

the traditional and painstaking approach of studying only one or two. And that leap forward is allowing us to determine more accurate biomarkers for aging, which will affect everything from when we need to start getting certain diagnostic tests to drug dosage.

THE UNPARALLELED POWER OF OMICS

One of the reasons we're able to make such great strides forward with research is that artificial intelligence allows us to process massive amounts of data.

We call this data *omics,* and it's transforming our ability to solve aging riddles that would otherwise take years if not decades to figure out. Instead of theorizing and setting out to find certain answers, we look at the data produced by the technology and find the answers there in an unbiased fashion.

Whole exome sequencing — the sequencing of the part of the genome made up of exons — is such an omic, where we have all the important sequences of most of the centenarians' genes that account for hundreds of millions of DNA letters multiplied by three thousand subjects. This is billions of data points, and we're asking the technology to tell us all the differences between the exomes of centenarians and their offspring and those of the control group. This narrows our search considerably, but there are still hundreds of thousands of differences in the DNA sequence between those with exceptional longevity and our control group. As a result, many of the points identified are going to be false positives, because if you have thousands of people in a study, some of the distinctions between the groups will occur just because of chance. That means some results may initially seem significant, but once we correct the results, not all of them will turn out to be statistically significant. At the same time, though, it's inevitable that we will eliminate some of the distinctions that actually *are* significant — in other words, false negatives, which are actually positive.

After correction, we still had about thirty thousand significant differences between centenarians and the control group, so we have assigned each of these differences to a pathway. This is important because it's less about what individual SNPs or variants do and more about what the pathways do. All the tens of thousands of differences are assigned to their own pathways, and now we're looking at the knowledge that we have from each pathway. And some of the pathways that are most significant are the signaling pathways for insulin, IGF, and mTOR. In other words, what we have learned from animal research lines up with these pathways. And thanks to Alan Shuldiner, vice president of Regeneron Pharmaceuticals, who performed the sequencing for free, we saved millions of dollars.

The technology that creates omics is also helping us to find longevity secrets that are hidden in proteins. In animal studies, we and other researchers learned that the blood of younger animals was somehow restoring youthfulness in older animals, but the question we needed to answer was which proteins were responsible for this "magic."

This is one of those questions that would have taken us a very long time to explore just a few years ago because we could only study several proteins at a time. But SomaLogic invented a method to measure five thousand proteins as quickly and accurately as we were able to measure one or two. Rather than measuring the proteins of centenarians, who are at the end of their lives, we wanted to find out first what the differences were between the centenarians' offspring and the control group. And thanks to Tony Wyss-Coray, one of SomaLogic's founders and a professor of neurology at

Stanford, we were able to look at these five thousand proteins in one thousand members of our LonGenity study, who are all age sixty-five to ninety-five. We examined if we could find proteins that could be biomarkers of aging. You can imagine that this is a huge amount of data, and because of Tony, what could have cost millions of dollars was done for us at no cost.

The technology identified 585 proteins whose levels increased or decreased significantly with age. So there are definitely proteins that are associated with biological age. And that's not even the best part of what we learned from the data. The results were so statistically significant that we know we can repeat this analysis many times and get the same results. To be classified as statistically significant, the probability value of a hypothesis — a measure of the probability of finding the same or more extreme results by chance — needs to be less than 0.005, and our results were between 10^{-40} and 10^{-80}. Adding to our excitement, some of the proteins that were identified are very large, and their levels increase severalfold with aging, so they are among the first we're studying.

We also found out that the five proteins we had previously identified as being most significant in terms of aging were barely significant compared with the top fifty that SomaLogic identified. And when we compared the results of the five hundred centenarians' offspring and the five hundred people in the control group, whose members were the same chronological age, we found something truly remarkable. The levels of only 235 of the 585 proteins changed significantly in the offspring, and this is because the offspring were biologically younger than the members of the control group. It's possible that if we retest them several years from now, the offspring will have just as many significant proteins as the control group, but for now, they are biologically younger. Not only that, but in the offspring, we found twenty-five proteins that are unique to them, and we think they may be protecting them from the hallmarks of aging. So far, we know that at least three of the proteins are protective. One of them, klotho, is typical in centenarians' offspring and not in the control group, and a company called Unity recently invested $250 million to commercialize this protein.

Many of the proteins associated with aging are the result of the breakdown of tissues, and we also see proteins that we and other researchers have linked with aging in longevity pathways such as GH/IGF-1. Many of these broken-down proteins may serve as excellent biological markers for the treatment of aging because if we succeed, the breakage should stop and we should see a decrease in the levels of these proteins. We want to see that the levels decrease with treatment before we embark on long, expensive studies that may not produce the effects we're hoping for.

And we are also working with Yale University pathologist Morgan Levine to create an instrument like a clock that will predict biological age based on a set of specific proteins. We expect it to be as good as or better than measuring methylation for estimating biological age. When we have standardized biomarkers for aging, we will need to show only the change in markers to get approval for a treatment instead of needing five years to show hard evidence. For example, no matter what method we use to lower cholesterol or blood pressure, we will prevent cardiovascular diseases, so aging will be about biomarkers that show change. The signature of our proteins that show biological age is, of course, much more predictive of mortality than the frailty index or chronological age.

PERSONALIZED MEDICINE

As genetic tests become more refined and less expensive, we can personalize medical treatments in ways that were not even conceivable in the past. This is one of the most exciting new frontiers because we know that the same drugs and treatments can have varying effects on men and women, young and old — there isn't any one thing that's good for everyone under all circumstances. But there may be drugs that target one hallmark of aging better than another.

We are also making advances in beginning to personalize diabetes treatments, and an NIH-funded study being conducted at several centers is exploring what the best treatments are for different people. So it won't be long before we will also be using personalized medicine to treat all the hallmarks of aging.

One of the best examples of personalized medicine already under way is the treatment for various types of cancer. Each type of cancer now has a different recommended treatment, and as research progresses, scientists will be able to customize these targeted approaches even more, which should lead to higher survival rates. One of the new immune treatment therapies is melanoma itself. My father may have unknowingly benefited from this approach long before it officially became a treatment.

When Dad was in his forties, he developed a persistent cough, and a chest x-ray showed a mass in his right lung that the radiologist suspected was a tumor. It was 1968, and surgeons in Israel did not have the capacity to perform this surgery, so he and my mother traveled to Sloan Kettering. I was thirteen at the time, and when he returned home, he looked fine. But one day soon after, he took me aside and said, "I don't know how much time I have to live, so I hope you will take care of your mother and sisters." He never offered information about a diagnosis or the surgery, so I didn't know why he suspected that his time might be coming to an end, but over the years, every now and again, he would give me this goodbye talk. After a while, I stopped believing that it was anything more than a father saying what he thought he should impart to his son.

It wasn't until I was a fellow at Sloan Kettering that the mystery was solved. As it turned out, my father's cancer was metastasis of melanoma that invaded most of his right lung and the chest cavity. His right lung had been surgically removed, and the surgeon removed all the cancer he could see in the chest cavity. It looked so bad that the surgeon didn't recommend follow-up treatment because he didn't think my father would live more than a few months. To everyone's surprise, he lived to be eighty-four years old, and when he did die, it was not from cancer. As it happens, one in one thousand people with melanoma have or develop an immunological capacity to deal with it. In my father's case, he must have had an ability to clear the cancer that was left after the surgery.

In the years to come, in addition to advanced technology — and also because of it — doctors will have much more information about their patients and aging in general. This will dramatically increase the accuracy of diagnoses and decrease the incidence of medical errors and negative drug interactions. Add those advantages to early detection, genetic testing, epigenetic assessment, aging clocks, personal health monitoring devices, and greater understanding of nutrition and exercise, and the result is decades more of good health and life.

ADVANCES IN EARLY DETECTION

We have a grant to identify the mechanism for resiliency to Alzheimer's disease in our centenarians, and we discovered they have a mutation in a gene called *ABCA1,* which is involved in a cholesterol disease called *Tangier.* It happens that ABCA1 is already a target for drug development to treat Alzheimer's, but we have other candidates as well.

At the same time, a member of our resiliency consortium, Catherine Kaczorowski, head of the Jackson Laboratory in Bar Harbor, Maine, a Nathan Shock Center of Excellence in the Basic Biology of Aging, is studying why some people who have a family history of Alzheimer's and brain changes associated with this disease do not lose their cognitive abilities. She's working to identify biomarkers of resilience that protect mice — including those that have a genetic predisposition for cognitive decline — from neurodegenerative diseases, including Alzheimer's. Rather than studying the factors that make mice and people susceptible to Alzheimer's, Kaczorowski is focused on finding the genetic and molecular mechanisms associated with the regulatory pathways that lead to resilience, and we're collaborating with her to make mice that are protected from Alzheimer's disease so she can study them. While this may sound far-fetched, the drug humanin has prevented age-related cognitive decline in mice, and there's good reason to believe it may benefit human cognition, too. You may recall that our centenarian Frieda had the highest humanin level on record, and she was mentally sharp long after she turned one hundred.

PIONEERING EXPLORATIONS

The race to find ways to keep people vital and healthy for as long as we live is inspiring scientists all over the world to explore uncharted territories with thousands of pursuits that may or may not pan out. I'm hopeful that some of their innovations will prove to be effective in double-blind clinical trials but until then, I'm sharing a few examples of ventures that I provided consultation for but have no financial stake in. I'm not yet convinced that they will change the face of aging, but I want to make the point that some of the "crazy" things being pursued might be crazy enough to work.

For example, in a relatively new realm of research, scientists are looking at how particular foods affect particular genes and other aspects of cell metabolism. There are also many biological extracts derived from plants — including metformin, which comes from the French lilac — that will be faster and easier to test because of new technology.

I suspect that nature has many potent forces that can be harnessed to target aging and associated diseases, and I'm betting that many of them will be totally unexpected. A company called Regenera Pharma is testing a botanical that appears to have helped animals and humans with a variety of age-related problems. Zadik Hazan, founder and chief scientific officer at Regenera, started the company with the mission to help people restore the function that's lost as a result of neurological diseases. We offered to test this drug at our center to see if it really targeted aging, and we couldn't demonstrate a significant effect on longevity, but we could show some other beneficial effects, such as reduced inflammation. Mice are not always great predictors of how a drug will work in people, though, and now Regenera has a leading drug candidate. This candidate, RPh201, is purified plant sap from the mastic gum plant, which is already being used in some foods and medicines. The drug is being tested for its regenerative activity and functional recovery benefits and has shown promising results in preclinical models and may have properties that protect against stroke, vascular dementia, and other neurological conditions. A double-blind study is under way to evaluate the effectiveness and safety of RPh201 in about 230 people who have been diagnosed with non-arteritic anterior ischemic optic neuropathy (NAION), which is a stroke of the optic nerve that impairs vision to the point of blindness. The participants will be studied to measure the drug's impact on visual function, so it will be a while before we know the results, but the potential is exciting.

There's also a lot of excitement around many innovative treatments that are being offered to slow and reverse the physical and cognitive decline currently associated with aging. For example, my rather recent mentor and friend Sami Sagol, who has studied the science of aging with great interest and invested in academia and the business of aging, invested in a hyperbaric center run by Shai Efrati, a smart and energetic doctor at Yitzhak Shamir Medical Center, in central Israel. Sami wanted to hear what I thought of this investment because of my understanding of aging and my training in hyperbaric medicine, which I received as an Israeli naval physician. He didn't realize when he approached me that my mother had been treated for deep infections with hyperbaric medicine and that some of my diabetic patients with infections had also benefited from this treatment. When diabetics with wounds are treated in hyperbaric chambers, the bacteria are exposed to oxygen and killed.

Sami's hoping that this therapy can also be beneficial for age-related diseases and particularly for cognitive decline. For the treatments at Shai's center, patients sit inside a chamber that looks like a submarine and is furnished like the business-class section of an airplane. They receive a high-oxygen treatment in a pressurized "cabin." The people who have started to have cognitive problems are treated weekly or biweekly for a few months, and they are reporting that they feel much better and that their cognitive functions are improving.

Shai says that by giving people nearly 100 percent oxygen under pressure, it can reach cells that oxygen doesn't often reach in older people. As we age, there are areas of the body, particularly the brain, that do not get enough blood supply and, therefore, not enough oxygen. If oxygen is successfully delivered to those areas, it can repair tissues and might even stimulate stem cells to initiate a process that's rejuvenating.

I can't help but be curious about whether

there is a strong placebo effect with the treatment, but the possibilities are worth more exploration. I look forward to the results of controlled studies that eliminate the placebo effect and test the effects of high and low doses of oxygen.

REVERSING CELLULAR AGE

In 1962, John B. Gurdon showed in a petri dish that cellular age could be reversed, and in 2006, Shinya Yamanaka discovered that a particular set of four genes could reprogram adult cells to become immature cells that could in turn develop into any type of cell. He laid the groundwork for scientists to grow new blood cells tissues and organs that are already being transplanted into people. In 2012, Gurdon and Yamanaka were jointly awarded the Nobel Prize in Physiology or Medicine for their work.

The "Yamanaka factors" have profound implications for aging, but they're not something we can simply ingest. They need to be delivered directly to cells, and one of the ways this is done is by putting these factors' information on a virus — modulated to remove the harmful aspects — and directing the virus to attack the cell. The challenge with the Yamanaka factors is that one of them is highly carcinogenic, but my buddy David Sinclair, founder of Iduna, found that he can take an old cell and make it young again by using only the three factors that are not carcinogenic. He delivers those three factors with a virus to the crushed optic nerves of mice, and this restores partial eyesight to mice with previously nonresponsive optic nerves. The viruses infect the nerve cells and transcribe the three factors so that they change the cells into cells that behave like stem cells. The same procedure has reversed glaucoma in mice. This research has far-reaching implications for repairing crushed nerves all over the body, including the spine. And in the future, we may even have a virus that can rejuvenate all cells from time to time, which would mean staying healthy and young for an extraordinarily long time.

In the meantime, researchers are exploring drugs that can deactivate the harmful results of a certain type of virus that wreaks havoc as we age. People are often surprised to find out that much of our DNA is composed of the DNA of viruses that infiltrated our own DNA a very long time ago. The virus DNA, called *retrotransposons,* was integrated into DNA and caused horrific mutations, but it also helped to create more diversity within species.

It is believed that the diversity of dogs, a subspecies of the wolf, is due to the integration of viruses in wolves. Fortunately, those integrated viruses remain inactive and do not reproduce. But recent research by my friend John Sedivy, a molecular and cellular biologist at Brown University, and neurosurgeon Sanjay Gupta has shown that a virus transposon called *LINE-1* wakes up with aging and behaves like a live flu virus. Our immune systems recognize it as an invader and increase inflammation. Antiviral treatments, such as those administered to HIV patients, can quiet it down, and we've learned that LINE-1 is also kept silent by a stress response protein called *Sirtuin 6* (Sirt6), which also helps to repair DNA, maintain telomeres, and lower inflammation. The exciting part of this story is that researchers are working toward creating specific drugs with Sirt6 that can keep the LINE-1 silent throughout our lives.

GENETIC ENGINEERING

In the years to come, we will see a wide array of advancements in genetic engineering and with them a confounding number of ethical questions. One of the things we can already do in animals is replace the APOE4 gene with a mutation that protects them from Alzheimer's, and we will probably be able to do this in humans someday, but should we? If a woman is pregnant and genetic testing shows that her daughter will be born with the BRCA1 gene, the ability to have that gene removed or replaced could sound like the right thing to do. If we can manipulate genes in a way that will ensure good health, it will be beneficial for individuals, society, and the economy. But what about adding in genes that can make a child more athletic, more artistic, or more musical? What if there is a gene that will give a child a higher IQ? These are a few of the questions we will face in the future, and governments will need to create new laws and negotiate with each other to regulate genetic engineering. Otherwise, it could become an arms-race scenario, with each country attempting to out-engineer the others, except in this case they would be engineering people. My friend Jamie Metzl has explored some longevity possibilities like these in *Hacking Darwin*.

For now, our best bet and safest course of action is to charge ahead in our quest to develop drugs that temper or stop the activity of undesirable genes and mimic the actions of beneficial variations and mutations so that we can all be young until we die.

Our DNA blueprint to be young isn't harmed or diminished by age, so slowing aging is just the first step. In time, we should be able to stop certain aspects of aging and reverse others.

If that sounds like an impossible dream, here's something that might change your mind — the ability to reverse aging is already contained within the human body. If we take the sperm of a seventy-year-old man and the egg of a fifty-year-old woman, we can determine the age of the sperm and the egg, and those ages will be about the same chronological ages of the donors. But we know that if you fertilize the fifty-year-old egg with the seventy-year-old sperm, the new cells that divide and begin the life of the fetus start at *age zero.* This is one of the most stunning and promising discoveries for the science of longevity, and the race to unravel this mystery is well under way.

Tomorrow will be brighter and healthier!

ACKNOWLEDGMENTS

This book and my work would not have been possible without the scientists and wonderful volunteers who made our research possible — the centenarians, their offspring, and the people in our control groups. These volunteers agreed to be interviewed and allowed us to take blood samples and conduct a variety of tests, including MRIs of their brains and CT scans of their coronary arteries. Many of these volunteers participated in studies throughout the years, showing up rain or shine and are inspiring us all. It's a beautiful partnership and I wish them all extended health span. To the wonderful study team members who guide our participants, treat them kindly, and keep them informed, thank you!

When I built a nutritional village in South Africa in the early 1980s, I purchased many three-legged pots for cooking. The most important feature of the pot is that it has three legs, which provide maximum stability. Three legs have supported me in my journey — my family, my colleagues, and my friends — and there are three legs to my family as well. The first is my wife, Laura, the reason I came to the United States and my true partner in life, along with our wonderfully talented and public-spirited children, Maya and Ben, who have extended endless help with reviewing the manuscript and providing comments. Maya and Ben are just beginning their professional journeys, which I hope will be as exciting as mine, and even longer and healthier. The second leg of the family represents my parents, David and Drora, who taught me the value of family and gave me my "little" sisters, Osnat and Netta, who encourage and advise me daily, with unconditional love, from different time zones. The third leg is my extended family. I am grateful to my aunt, Ruti Barzilai, now the matriarch of our family; to my brothers-in-law and sisters-in-law; to Ayal and Orna Bar-David; and to Bernice and Jerry Rubenstein, who have supported my journey in so many ways. I am inspired by my nieces and nephews, whom I hope will benefit from the ongoing research in the field of aging.

Many of my colleagues are mentioned throughout the manuscript, but there are many others who made amazing contributions to the field or have collaborated with me during my thirty-year journey. My first mentor is my father, David, whose experience as an internist, an endocrinologist, a chief of medicine, and dean of a medical school is always on my mind. He and my uncle Ami were medical pioneers in Israel and both were inspirations to me.

I owe special thanks to three people who have been essential threads in the fabric of my personal and professional life: Hassy Cohen, my partner in science, biotech, and friendship for more than forty years; Jon Stern, who has been like a brother to me for decades and has taught me entrepreneurship; and David Sinclair, a friend and partner in many efforts, whose science inspires me and the entire geoscience field. Other scientists who opened the most important doors at crucial times in my career and allowed me to become a leader include Eddy Karnieli, Ralph deFronzo, Paul Deuitch, Amir Lerman, Norman Fleischer, Harry Shamoon, Luciano Rossetti, George Martin, Alan Shuldiner, Felipe Sierra, Ron Kohansky, Jill Crandall, Meredith Hawkins, John Amatruda, Jeff Pessin,

Joe Verghese, Yousin Suh, and Gil Atzmon.

Albert Einstein College of Medicine has been my professional home for nearly three decades and was supportive of what may have seemed at the time a crazy idea to open the Institute for Aging Research. This institute could not exist without the strong leadership of partners I admire, my friends and collaborators Ana Maria Cuervo and Jan Vijg. The people I have trained at Einstein have made me wiser and my research could not have progressed without them. Among many trainees, I am particularly proud of Sofiya Milman, who is now advancing the SuperAgers studies; and Derek Huffman, who is advancing discoveries in models of aging. Together with Zhengdong Zhang, Fernando Macian, Rajath Singh, Dengshong Cai, and others, they are the future leaders of the institute and I know our pending health span is in good hands.

I am also indebted to the American Federation of Aging Research (AFAR), which provided me with research funding in the very early stages of my career. AFAR is an exemplary nonprofit organization that leads current efforts in assuring the development of the therapeutic pipeline by funding aging research and is overseeing the funding and operation of TAME. I thank my AFAR colleagues, Stephanie Lederman, Odette van der Willik, and the board members and staff of AFAR.

Through my work and involvement with AFAR, other leaders who joined with me to spread the message of geroscience and became my friends during the journey include Steven Austed, James Kirkland, Anrzej Bartke, Tom Kirkwood, Jay Olshansky, Brian Kennedy, Rafa de Cabo, Yap Seng Chong, Judy Campisi, Joan Mannick, Vera Gorbunova, Steve Horvath, Morgan Levine, Arlan Richardson, Peter Rabinovitch, Andrei Gudkov, Tom Rando, Tony Wyss-Coray, Laura Niedernhofer, Paul Robbins, Tom Perls, Paola Sebastiani, Luigi Ferrucci, Rafa de Cabo, and other members of the Nathan Shock Center of Excellence, the Paul F. Glenn Center for Biology of Aging Research, and the Dorot Foundation.

AFAR also coordinates the TAME effort led by a bunch of scientists that spent a lot of time that was not funded. I am most indebted to Steve Kritchevsky, Mark Espeland, and Jaimie Justice, who did so much heavy lifting, and the other members of our executive committee, Vanita Aroda, George Kuchel, and Judy Bahnson. There are fourteen centers for TAME led by distinct leaders: Thomas Gill, Beth Lewis, Claudine

George, Marco Pahor, Hermes Florez, Anne Newman, Rina Wing, Larry Apple, Karen Margolis, and Mary McDermott. Thank you all for volunteering your time to make a template for this and other studies. Your efforts will prove our geroscience concepts, will probably save trillions of dollars in medical costs, and will change our lives.

My work has also taken me outside of the field of science and, as a result, I have made many new friends who have been very influential and supportive. Sami Sagol, who financially supports academic research and companies focusing on health span and encourages his network to support them, too, is determined to stay young and promised to give my eulogy, although he is more than a decade older than me. Jim Mellon is inspiring the field and has become a friend, a partner for many activities, and someone whose advice I value. Jamie Metzl is a Renaissance man, an adviser, a believer, and a very dear friend. Sergey Young and James Peyer are devoted to TAME and bring a wealth of knowledge and insight. Albion Fitzgerald is a unique and outstanding angel who has led CohBar steadfastly. My life also is enriched by my interactions with Mehmood Khan, David Setboun, Mark Collins, Tristan Edwards, Tom Kahn, Ron

Kahn, Gabi Barbash, Zan Alexander, Peter Attia, Ilia Stambler, Tina Woods, and Oren Vanek.

The actual writing of this book involved several dedicated professionals. I am grateful to my literary agent, Melissa Flashman at Janklow & Nesbit Associates, for opening the door for this opportunity and teaching me the publishing ropes and to my editor, Elizabeth Beier, and assistant editor Hannah Phillips at St. Martin's Press for their editorial insight and guidance. But, most of all, I am indebted to my coauthor, Toni Robino and my editor, Doug Wagner of Windword Literary Services. Many people ask how this book came to be, given that English is not my first language and my written words often show that. Toni read and listened to my words and then "translated" them into what you see on these pages and Doug had our backs on every page. I could not have done this without them. They worked tirelessly while being so kind and flexible and making this journey a pleasure every step of the way.

ABOUT THE AUTHOR

Nir Barzilai, M.D., is the founding Director of the Institute for Aging Research at Albert Einstein College of Medicine and the Nathan Shock Center for Excellence in the Basic Biology of Aging, and discovered the first longevity gene in humans. He is also the director of the Diabetes Research and Training Center Physiology Core and the co-director of the Montefiore Hospital Diabetes Clinic.

The employees of Thorndike Press hope you have enjoyed this Large Print book. All our Thorndike, Wheeler, and Kennebec Large Print titles are designed for easy reading, and all our books are made to last. Other Thorndike Press Large Print books are available at your library, through selected bookstores, or directly from us.

For information about titles, please call:
   (800) 223-1244

or visit our website at:
   gale.com/thorndike

To share your comments, please write:
   Publisher
   Thorndike Press
   10 Water St., Suite 310
   Waterville, ME 04901